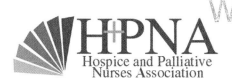

Hospice and Palliative
Nurses Association

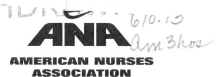

AMERICAN NURSES
ASSOCIATION

*H*OSPICE AND *P*ALLIATIVE *N*URSING:

*S*COPE AND *S*TANDARDS

OF *P*RACTICE

nurses
books
.org

The Publishing Program of ANA

HOSPICE AND PALLIATIVE NURSES ASSOCIATION
AMERICAN NURSES ASSOCIATION
SILVER SPRING, MARYLAND
2007

Library of Congress Cataloging-in-Publication data

Hospice and Palliative Nurses Association.

Hospice and palliative nursing : scope and standards of practice / Hospice and Palliative Nurses Association [and] American Nurses Association. — [4th ed.]
p. ; cm.

Rev. ed. of: Scope and standards of hospice and palliative nursing practice / Hospice and Palliative Nurses Association, American Nurses Association [3rd ed.]. c2002.

Includes bibliographical references and index.
ISBN-13: 978-1-55810-253-8 (pbk.)
ISBN-10: 1-55810-253-1 (pbk.)
1. Hospice care—Standards—United States. 2. Terminal care—Standards—United States. 3. Palliative treatment—Standards—United States. 4. Nursing—Standards—United States.
I. American Nurses Association. II. Scope and standards of hospice and palliative nursing practice. III. Title.

[DNLM: 1. Hospice Care—standards—United States—Practice Guideline. 2. Nursing Care—standards—United States—Practice Guideline. 3. Palliative Care—standards—United States—Practice Guideline. WY 152 H828h 2007]

RT87.T45H64 2007
616′.029—dc22   2007020978

The American Nurses Association (ANA) is a national professional association. This ANA publication—*Hospice and Palliative Nursing: Scope and Standards of Practice*—reflects the thinking of the nursing profession on various issues and should be reviewed in conjunction with state board of nursing policies and practices. State law, rules, and regulations govern the practice of nursing, while *Hospice and Palliative Nursing: Scope and Standards of Practice* guides nurses in the application of their professional skills and responsibilities.

The Hospice and Palliative Nurses Association (HPNA) is a membership organization for individual members of the nursing team working in the specialty of hospice and palliative care across the life span continuum. Guided by its mission of promoting excellence in end-of-life nursing**,** HPNA has become the nationally recognized organization providing resources and support for advanced practice nurses, registered nurses, licensed practical nurses, and nursing assistants who care for people with life-limiting and terminal illness.

Published by Nursesbooks.org
The Publishing Program of ANA

American Nurses Association
8515 Georgia Avenue, Suite 400
Silver Spring, MD 20910-3492
1-800-274-4ANA
http://www.nursesbooks.org/

ANA is the only full-service professional organization representing the nation's 2.9 million Registered Nurses through its 54 constituent member associations. ANA advances the nursing profession by fostering high standards of nursing practice, promoting the economic and general welfare of nurses in the workplace, projecting a positive and realistic view of nursing, and lobbying the Congress and regulatory agencies on healthcare issues affecting nurses and the public.

Development of these standards was made possible in part by a grant from New York University and Project Death in America.

Design: Scott Bell, Arlington, VA; Freedom by Design, Alexandria, VA; Stacy Maguire, Sterling, VA ~ *Editing & indexing*: Steven A. Jent, Denton, TX ~ *Proofreading*: Lisa Munsat Anthony, Chapel Hill, NC ~ *Composition*: House of Equations, Inc., Arden, NC ~ *Printing*: McArdle Printing, Upper Marlboro, MD

First printing July 2007.

ISBN-13: 978-1-55810-253-8   ISBN-10: 1-55810-253-1   SAN: 851-3481   2.5M   07/07

CONTRIBUTORS

Editors

Constance Dahlin, MSN, APRN, BC-PCM
Elaine Glass, MSN, APRN, BC-PCM

Reviewers

Dena Jean Sutermaster, RN, MSN, CHPN®
Judy Lentz, RN, MSN, NHA

ANA Staff

Carol J. Bickford, PhD, RN, BC—Content editor
Yvonne Daley Humes, MSA—Project coordinator
Matthew Seiler, RN, Esq.—Legal counsel

CONTENTS

Preface

Statement on the Scope and Standards of Hospice and Palliative Nursing

This document, developed by the Hospice and Palliative Nurses Association, is the fourth edition and represents the cumulative revision of the three previous editions. The first edition, in 1987, focused on basic hospice nursing. The second, in 2000, brought together hospice and palliative care. In 2002, the third edition described the evolution of this specialty nursing practice by addressing both generalist and advanced practice hospice and palliative nursing. This fourth edition is an expansion of the third edition within the American Nurses Association framework.

The hope of the Hospice and Palliative Nurses Association is that these standards will help to further advance the practice of hospice and palliative care and to set benchmarks for all registered nurses and advanced practice nurses who practice nursing within the realm of life-limiting, progressive illness or end-of-life care.

Introduction

By developing and then articulating the scope and standards of professional nursing practice, the specialty of hospice and palliative nursing informs society about the parameters of nursing practice and guides the formulation of rules and regulations that determine hospice and palliative nursing practice. However, because each state creates its own laws and regulations governing nursing, the designated limits, functions, and titles for nurses, especially those in advanced practice, may vary significantly from state to state. As in all nursing specialties, hospice and palliative nurses must accept professional practice accountability and ensure that their practice remains within the scope of their state nurse practice act, professional code of ethics, and professional practice standards.

Because life-limiting illness increases dramatically with age, hospice and palliative nurses often focus on the care of older adults. The management of these older adults requires special skills.

Nursing practice is differentiated according to the nurse's educational preparation and level of practice. A number of undergraduate programs include coursework in hospice and palliative care. Some graduate nursing programs permit specialization in palliative care; others offer post-master's degree certificates in this area. The hospice and palliative nurse may practice from a generalist through advanced level of competency. In this document, the title Advanced Practice Registered Nurse (APRN) is used as an inclusive term to describe the common core of knowledge, skills, and abilities of both the clinical nurse specialist (CNS) and the nurse practitioner (NP). The advanced practice hospice and palliative nurse demonstrates such advanced competencies to promote the quality of life for individuals and their families experiencing life-limiting, progressive illness. Nursing role specialties include hospice and palliative care case managers and nursing administrators at the executive and manager levels.

The goal of palliative care is to promote the best possible quality of life for patients and families so that they may live as fully and comfortably as possible. Palliative care recognizes dying as part of the normal process of living and focuses on maintaining the quality of remaining life. Palliative care affirms life and neither hastens nor postpones death.

Palliative care exists in the hope and belief that through appropriate care and the promotion of a caring community, sensitive to their needs, patients and their families may be free to attain a degree of mental, emotional, and spiritual preparation for death that is satisfactory to them. Although palliative care has no current regulatory time restrictions, hospice care is the final portion of the palliative care continuum regulated by Medicare as a 6-month period if the illness runs its normal course.

Evolution of Hospice and Palliative Nursing

The landmark SUPPORT study (Study to Understand Prognoses and Preferences for Outcomes and Risk of Treatment) by Knaus et al. (1995) highlighted an urgent need for healthcare professionals prepared and committed to improving the quality of life for seriously ill and dying patients and their families. These researchers conducted a two-year prospective observational study with 4,301 patients from teaching hospitals in the United States, followed by a two-year controlled clinical trial with 4,804 patients and their physicians who were randomized either to a control group or to an intervention group that received educational information related to the end of life. Despite the SUPPORT intervention, the study found:

- a continued lack of communication between patients and their physician providers, particularly related to end-of-life preferences,
- an aggressiveness of medical treatments, and
- a high level of pain reported by seriously ill and dying patients.

Knaus et al. believe that improving the experience of seriously ill and dying patients requires an individual and collective commitment of healthcare providers as well as proactive efforts at shaping the caregiving process. Having invested 28 million dollars in the SUPPORT study, the Robert Wood Johnson Foundation (RWJF) has extended its commitment to end-of-life care, recognizing the "overriding need to change the kind of care dying Americans receive" (Last Acts Task Force, 1998).

Educational preparation for end-of-life care has been inconsistent at best and neglected for the most part, in both undergraduate and graduate curricula (AACN, 1997). In accordance with the International Council of Nurses mandate that nurses have a unique and primary responsibility for ensuring the peaceful death of patients, the American Association of Colleges of Nursing (AACN), supported by RWJF, convened a round table of expert nurses to discuss and initiate educational change related to palliative care. These nurse experts concluded that the precepts of hospice care are essential principles for all end-of-life care, and include the following assumptions:

- Persons are living until the moment of death.
- Coordinated care should be offered by a variety of professionals with attention to the physical, psychological, social, and spiritual needs of patients and their families.
- Care should be sensitive to patient and family diversity.

The group proposed that these precepts be added to the foundational content in the education of nurses. The resulting document, "Peaceful Death," outlined baccalaureate competencies for palliative and hospice care and the content areas in which these competencies can be taught (AACN, 1997).

To emphasize the role of nursing in end-of-life care, the American Nurses Association (ANA) issued a position statement regarding the promotion of comfort and relief of pain of dying patients (ANA, 2003). This statement reinforces the nurse's obligation to promote comfort and to ensure aggressive efforts to relieve pain and suffering. Initiatives are underway in nursing to include palliative care content in licensing examinations and to revise nursing textbooks to address palliative care. Specialized palliative care educational initiatives have been offered in the last five years, such as the End-of-life Nursing Education Consortium (ELNEC). ELNEC is supported by a major grant from RWJF to AACN and City of Hope National Medical Center (AACN & CHNMC, 2005).

One goal of undergraduate ELNEC was to train 1,000 nurse educators from associate degree and baccalaureate programs in end-of-life care. Another cohort was to focus on teaching faculty at graduate programs; over 300 graduate program faculty have attended this curriculum. Another program has educated 206 oncology nurses. Pediatric ELNEC faculty members have educated 400 nurses and a new curriculum will focus on end-of-life care in the critical care setting. ELNEC-Geriatrics programs began in February of 2007. The course includes essential content for the highest quality end-of-life geriatric care and is open to long-term-care nurses and hospice nurses who serve patients in long-term care.

In 2004, the National Consensus Project (NCP) published *Clinical Practice Guidelines for Quality Palliative Care,* commonly referred to as the *NCP Guidelines*. These guidelines have been endorsed by numerous medical and nursing specialty groups, and encompass populations of all ages. More importantly, the NCP Guidelines served as the foundation of the *National Quality Forum Framework for Preferred Practices for Palliative and Hospice Care,* scheduled to be published in 2007.

National, state, and local indicators point to the need to prepare APRNs who have advanced knowledge and skill in hospice and palliative care, are competent to provide patient care across the life span, and can assume leadership roles in a variety of settings. APRNs can play a vital role in palliative care by assessing, implementing, coordinating, and evaluating care throughout the course of the illness, as well as by counseling and educating patients and families and facilitating continuity of care between hospital and home. Because of their proximity to patients, APRNs are in an ideal position to assess, diagnose, and treat pain and other symptoms. APRNs also identify ethical issues facing individuals and families, develop strategies to assist them in defining expected goals of care, and access and coordinate appropriate care.

Palliative care is a rapidly developing specialty in health care. In September 2006, the American Board of Medical Specialties (ABMS) voted to make hospice and palliative medicine an ABMS subspecialty. Hospice and palliative care services are being developed across the country, including inpatient palliative and hospice units, consultations teams, community or home hospice programs, ambulatory palliative care programs, and programs in skilled nursing facilities. Current estimates are that 30% of hospitals have inpatient palliative care programs (CAPC, 2006).

Professional Association and Certification

In 1987, the Hospice Nurses Association (HNA) was formed. This group became the first professional organization dedicated to promoting excellence in the practice of hospice nursing. Consistent with that goal, the HNA Board of Directors appointed the National Board for the Certification of Hospice Nurses (NBCHN) in 1992. In March of 1994, NBCHN offered the first certification examination and the credential of Certified Registered Nurse Hospice (CRNH).

In 1997, recognizing the similarity in the nursing practice of the hospice nurse and the palliative nurse, HNA expanded to embrace palliative nursing practice and became the Hospice and Palliative Nurses Association (HPNA). Hospice and palliative nurses were providing patient and family care in more diverse settings and the fundamental nursing concepts developed in hospices were being applied to other practice environments. The results of the 1998 Role Delineation Study, repeated in 2006, commissioned by NBCHN, revealed only minor differences in practice between end-of-life care offered by hospice nurses and palliative nurses working in non-hospice settings. These differences correlated with requirements of the role or practice setting.

In 1999, NBCHN became the National Board for the Certification of Hospice and Palliative Nurses (NBCHPN®), offering a new professional certification designation to recognize basic competence in hospice and palliative nursing—Certified Hospice and Palliative Nurse (CHPN®), thereby retiring the CRNH credential. In 2004, certification was also offered to APRNs to acknowledge their expertise in palliative care. These were first designated as APRN, BC-PCM. However, with the sole proprietorship of the exam, NBCHPN retired that credential and now APRNs are ACHPNs®. Currently, there are 271 APRNs certified in palliative care.

By 2007, the number of credentialed registered nurses had risen to over 10,000. As demographics change and advanced illnesses and end-of-life needs increase, NBCHPN continues to provide assurance of competency of both generalist and advanced practice registered hospice and palliative nurses who administer care by strengthening the *Scope and Standards of Hospice and Palliative Nursing Practice.*

SCOPE OF HOSPICE AND PALLIATIVE NURSING PRACTICE

The scope of practice of hospice and palliative nursing continues to evolve as the science and art of palliative care develops. Hospice and palliative nursing reflects a holistic philosophy of care implemented across the life span and across diverse health settings. In a matrix of affiliation, including the patient and family and other members of the interdisciplinary care team, hospice and palliative nurses provide evidence-based physical, emotional, psychosocial, and spiritual or existential care to individuals and families experiencing life-limiting, progressive illness. The goal of hospice and palliative nursing is to promote and improve the patient's quality of life through the relief of suffering along the course of illness, through the death of the patient, and into the bereavement period of the family. This goal is enhanced by the following activities:

- Comprehensive history: chief complaint, history of present illness, medical and surgical history, family history, social history, immunization history, and allergies

- Review of systems and associated pain and symptoms

- Comprehensive physical and mental status examinations

- Determination of functional status

- Identification of developmental needs for all age groups

- Procurement of appropriate laboratory data and diagnostic studies or procedures

- Determination of effective and ineffective pharmacologic and non-pharmacologic therapies for symptom management

- Identification of past and present goals of care as stated by patient, surrogate, or healthcare proxy or as documented through advanced care planning

- Identification of health beliefs, values, and practices as related to culture, ethnicity, and religion or spirituality

- Recognition of response to advanced illness

- Determination of emotional status such as normal versus complicated grief, depression, anxiety, agitation, and terminal restlessness

- Identification of individual–family communication and coping patterns—past and present
- Assessment of patient and family support systems and environmental risks
- Determination of patient and family financial resources
- Assessment of spiritual needs, including meaning of life, illness, and death, as well as a sense of hope or hopelessness, a need for forgiveness, fears, and a connectedness to self, others, nature, and God or a Higher Being

Hospice and palliative care is provided to patients of all ages across the continuum of care from acute care to community care, recognizing that older adults comprise the predominant patient group. Of the 15 leading causes of death, over half are the predominant cause of death in older adults. As with the elderly who are both seriously ill and of limited decision-making capacity, parents or guardians have the responsibility to make the healthcare decisions for their child. This can create significant tensions as the older child is able to become a meaningful participant in care decisions.

Clinical Practice Setting

Practice settings for hospice and palliative nursing are changing in response to the dynamic nature of today's healthcare environment. Hospice and palliative nursing is provided for patients and their families in a variety of care locations including, but not limited to:

- Acute care hospital units
- Long-term-care facilities
- Rehabilitation facilities, assisted living facilities
- Inpatient, home, or residential hospices
- Palliative care clinics or ambulatory settings
- Private practices
- Veterans facilities
- Corrections facilities

Levels of Hospice and Palliative Nursing Practice

Hospice and palliative nurses are licensed registered nurses who are educationally prepared in nursing. Hospice and palliative nurses are qualified for specialty practice at two levels: generalist and advanced. These levels are differentiated by education, complexity of practice, and performance of certain nursing functions.

Generalist Level of Hospice and Palliative Nursing Practice

Registered nurses at the generalist level have completed a nursing program and passed the state licensure examination for registered nurses. Registered nurses who practice in hospice and palliative care settings may provide direct patient and family care or function as educators, case managers, nurse clinicians, administrators, and other nursing roles. Their practice should reflect the scope and standards of hospice and palliative nursing delineated in this document.

The generalist competencies in hospice and palliative care, summarized below, represent the knowledge, skills, and abilities demonstrated when providing evidence-based physical, emotional, psychosocial, and spiritual care (HPNA, 2001, 2002). The care is provided in a collaborative manner across the life span in diverse settings to individuals and families experiencing life-limiting, progressive illness.

Clinical Judgment

The hospice and palliative nurse demonstrates critical thinking, analysis, and clinical judgment in all aspects of hospice and palliative care for patients and families experiencing life-limiting illness. This includes use of the nursing process to address the physical, psychosocial, and spiritual needs of patients and families. The generalist and the advanced practice hospice and palliative nurse must respond to all disease processes, including, but not limited to, neurological, cardiac, pulmonary, oncology, renal, hepatic dementias, diabetes, and HIV/AIDS. Clinical judgment is demonstrated in providing effective pain and symptom management.

Advocacy and Ethics

The hospice and palliative nurse incorporates ethical principles and professional standards in the care of patients and families experiencing life-limiting, progressive illnesses. The nurse identifies and advocates for the wishes and preferences of the patient and patient's family, promotes ethical and legal decision making, and improves access to care and community resources by influencing or formulating health and social policy.

Professionalism

The hospice and palliative nurse exhibits knowledge, attitude, behavior, and skills that are consistent with the professional standards, code of ethics, and scope of practice for hospice and palliative nursing. Examples of professionalism include:

- Contributing to improved quality and cost-effective hospice and palliative services.
- Participating in the generation, testing, and evaluation of hospice and palliative care knowledge and practice.
- Participating in the hospice and palliative care organizations.

Collaboration

The hospice and palliative nurse actively promotes dialogue and collaboration with patients and families and facilitates collaborative practice with the healthcare team and community to address and plan for issues related to living with and dying from chronic, life-limiting, progressive illnesses through the bereavement phase.

Systems Thinking

The hospice and palliative nurse identifies and utilizes the system resources necessary to enhance the quality of life for patients and families experiencing life-limiting, progressive illnesses through knowledge and negotiation.

Cultural Competence

The hospice and palliative nurse respects and honors the diversity and unique characteristics of patients, families, and colleagues in hospice and palliative care and bereavement. Cultural competence also means that hospice and palliative nurses address the psychosocial and spiritual needs of patients and families throughout the dying process and bereavement. Cultural values and attitudes are incorporated into the plans of care throughout the continuum.

Facilitation of Learning

The hospice and palliative nurse promotes the learning of patient, family, self, members of the healthcare team, and the community by developing, implementing, and evaluating formal and informal education related to living with, and dying from, life-limiting progressive illnesses. This includes creating a healing environment that promotes and permits a peaceful death. The nurse creates opportunities and initiatives for hospice and palliative care education for patients, families, colleagues, and community as well.

Communication

The hospice and palliative nurse uses effective verbal, nonverbal, and written communication with patients and families, members of the healthcare team, and the community at large in order to therapeutically address and accurately convey the hospice and palliative care needs of patients and families throughout the disease process and bereavement. Communication at the generalist level includes using therapeutic communication skills in all interactions throughout the palliative care continuum.

Advanced Practice Level of Hospice and Palliative Nursing Practice

Advanced practice hospice and palliative nursing is an emerging role that responds to the individual, professional, and societal needs related to the experience of life-limiting, progressive illness. The advanced practice hospice and palliative registered nurse is a registered nurse (RN) educated at the master's level or higher in nursing as a clinical nurse specialist (CNS) or nurse practitioner (NP). An advanced practice hospice and palliative registered nurse has the knowledge, skills, and abilities to perform all aspects of basic hospice and palliative nursing as well as to assume the responsibilities of advanced-level care. Advanced practice hospice and palliative registered nurses are distinguished by their ability to synthesize complex data, implement advanced plans of care, and provide leadership in hospice and palliative care. The roles of advanced practice hospice and palliative registered nurses include, but are not limited to:

- Expert clinician
- Leader and facilitator of interdisciplinary teams

- Educator
- Researcher
- Consultant
- Collaborator
- Advocate
- Case manager
- Administrator

Advanced practice hospice and palliative nurses who have fulfilled the requirements established by their state nurse practice acts may be authorized to assume autonomous responsibility for clinical role functions, which may include prescription of controlled substances, medications, or therapies. To practice as an advanced practice hospice and palliative registered nurse, national certification in advanced practice hospice and palliative nursing is recommended. The advanced practice hospice and palliative registered nurse may have concurrent advanced practice certification in another specialty as well.

STANDARDS OF HOSPICE AND PALLIATIVE NURSING PRACTICE

The standards of hospice and palliative nursing practice are authoritative statements established by the Hospice and Palliative Nurses Association for the nursing profession and the public. The standards identify the responsibilities for which hospice and palliative nurses are accountable. The standards reflect the values and priorities of hospice and palliative nursing and provide a framework for the evaluation of practice. The standards are written in measurable terms and define hospice and palliative nurses' accountability to the public and describe the patient and family outcomes for which they are responsible.

The standards are divided into two sections: the Standards of Practice and the Standards of Professional Performance. Each section identifies criteria that allow the standards to be measured. The criteria include key indicators of competent practice. The standards remain stable over time as they reflect the philosophical values of the profession. However, the criteria should be revised to incorporate advancements in scientific knowledge, technology, and clinical practice. The criteria must be consistent with current nursing practice and reflect evidence-based practice.

Standards of Practice

Standards of practice describe a competent level of generalist and advanced practice registered nursing care, as demonstrated by the nursing process:

- Assessment
- Diagnosis
- Outcomes identification
- Planning
- Implementation (coordination of care, health teaching and health promotion, consultation, and prescriptive authority and treatment)
- Evaluation

The development and maintenance of a therapeutic nurse–patient and family relationship is essential throughout the nursing process. The nursing process forms the foundation of clinical decision making and encompasses all significant actions taken by hospice and palliative nurses in providing care to individuals and families. Several recurrent themes of nursing practice require attention:

- Providing age-appropriate, culturally, ethnically, and spiritually sensitive care and support

- Maintaining a safe environment

- Educating patients and families to identify appropriate settings and treatment options

- Assuring continuity of care and transitioning to the next appropriate setting

- Coordinating care across settings and among caregivers

- Managing information and protecting confidentiality

- Communicating promptly and effectively

A fundamental practice focus for hospice and palliative care is the plan of care, which is developed with the patient and family (with them as the center of care) and the interdisciplinary team in all practice activities. At the very minimum, the interdisciplinary team must include the physician, the nurse, the social worker, and clergy. Care responsibilities extend beyond the death of the patient to include a minimum of at least a year for bereavement care.

In addition to the distinct levels of nursing care—generalist and advanced—hospice and palliative nurses fulfill other roles. The nursing role specialty most prominent in hospice and palliative nursing is the hospice and palliative case manager. The case manager facilitates the activities of the interdisciplinary team within the regulatory requirements published as the Conditions of Participation as defined by the Health and Human Services Department. Specific criteria are included in this document to address the standards of practice of this role.

Standards of Professional Performance

Standards of professional performance and the associated measurement criteria describe competent professional role behaviors, including activities related to:

- Quality of practice
- Education
- Professional practice evaluation
- Collegiality
- Collaboration
- Ethics
- Research
- Resource utilization
- Leadership

Hospice and palliative nurses must be self-directed and purposeful in seeking necessary knowledge and skills to develop and maintain their competency. Hospice and palliative nurses' professionalism is enhanced through membership in their professional organizations, certification in their specialty, and professional development through academic and continuing education.

STANDARDS OF HOSPICE AND PALLIATIVE NURSING PRACTICE

STANDARDS OF PRACTICE

STANDARD 1. ASSESSMENT

The hospice and palliative registered nurse collects comprehensive data pertinent to the patient's health or the situation.

Measurement Criteria:

The hospice and palliative registered nurse:

- Collects data in a systematic and ongoing process using critical thinking, analysis, and judgment.

- Involves the patient, family, other healthcare providers, and environment, as appropriate, in holistic data collection.

- Prioritizes data collection activities based on the patient's immediate condition or anticipated needs of the patient, the family, or the situation.

- Adapts assessment techniques to address the differing physiological and psychosocial characteristics of older and younger patients.

- Uses appropriate evidence-based assessment and research techniques and instruments in collecting pertinent data.

- Uses analytical models and problem-solving tools.

- Synthesizes available data, information, and knowledge relevant to the situation to identify patterns and variances.

- Documents relevant data in an organized and retrievable format.

- Communicates to other interdisciplinary team members and consultants.

Continued ▶

Additional Measurement Criteria for the Advanced Practice Hospice and Palliative Registered Nurse:

The advanced practice hospice and palliative registered nurse:

- Prescribes and interprets diagnostic tests and procedures relevant to the patient's current status.

- Organizes family meetings to determine the patient's and family members' wishes and preferences and to identify areas of conflict, agreement, and understanding among each other and with the healthcare team.

- Reviews allergies and current medications for maximum effectiveness and possible need for adjustment based on further assessments.

Standard 2. Diagnosis
The hospice and palliative registered nurse analyzes the assessment data to determine nursing diagnoses or issues.

Measurement Criteria:

The hospice and palliative registered nurse:

- Derives the nursing diagnoses or issues based on assessment data, which includes actual or potential responses to alterations in health.

- Validates the nursing diagnoses or issues with the patient, the family, and the interdisciplinary team as well as other healthcare providers when possible and appropriate.

- Recognizes the influence of age on the patient's condition when formulating nursing diagnoses.

- Documents nursing diagnoses or issues in a manner that facilitates the determination of the expected outcomes and plan of care.

- Communicates to other interdisciplinary team members or consultants.

Additional Measurement Criteria for the Advanced Practice Hospice and Palliative Registered Nurse:

The advanced practice hospice and palliative registered nurse:

- Systematically compares and contrasts clinical findings with normal and abnormal variations and developmental events in formulating a differential diagnosis.

- Utilizes complex data and information obtained during interview, examination, diagnostic procedures, and family meetings in identifying nursing diagnoses.

- Assists staff in developing and maintaining competency in the diagnostic process.

STANDARD 3. OUTCOMES IDENTIFICATION

The hospice and palliative registered nurse, in partnership with the interdisciplinary healthcare team, identifies expected outcomes for a plan of care individualized to the patient or the situation.

Measurement Criteria:

The hospice and palliative registered nurse:

- Involves the patient, family, interdisciplinary team, and other healthcare providers in formulating expected outcomes to improve quality of life.

- Derives age- and culturally appropriate expected outcomes from the nursing diagnoses.

- Considers associated risks, benefits, costs, current scientific evidence, and clinical expertise when formulating expected outcomes.

- Defines expected outcomes in terms of the patient's and family's goals of care, the patient's values, ethical considerations, environment, or situation, with such consideration as associated risks, benefits and costs, and current scientific evidence.

- Includes a time estimate for attainment of expected outcomes.

- Develops expected outcomes that provide direction for continuity of care across care settings and through the family bereavement.

- Modifies expected outcomes based on changes in the status of the patient or evaluation of the situation.

- Documents expected outcomes as measurable goals.

- Communicates to other interdisciplinary team members and consultants.

Additional Measurement Criteria for the Advanced Practice Hospice and Palliative Registered Nurse:

The advanced practice hospice and palliative registered nurse:

- Identifies expected outcomes that incorporate scientific evidence and are achievable through implementation of evidence-based practices.

- Conducts family meetings periodically to clarify and reaffirm the goals of care.

- Identifies expected outcomes that incorporate both cost and clinical effectiveness, patient satisfaction, and continuity and consistency among providers.

- Supports the use of clinical guidelines linked to positive patient outcomes.

- Utilizes the knowledge that expected outcomes in older adults often differ from outcomes among younger individuals and pediatric patients.

STANDARD 4. PLANNING

The hospice and palliative registered nurse develops a plan of care that prescribes strategies and alternatives to attain expected outcomes.

Measurement Criteria:

The hospice and palliative registered nurse:

- Promotes the patient's power of choice in decision making.

- Develops an individualized plan of care that considers patient characteristics or the situation (e.g., age- and culturally appropriate, environmentally sensitive).

- Develops the plan of care negotiated in conjunction with the patient, family, interdisciplinary team, and others, as appropriate.

- Includes strategies within the plan of care that address each of the identified nursing diagnoses or issues, which may include strategies for promotion and restoration of health and prevention of illness, injury, and disease.

- Provides for continuity within the plan of care across settings and through the family bereavement.

- Incorporates an implementation pathway or timeline within the plan of care.

- Establishes priorities within the plan of care with the patient, family, interdisciplinary team, and others as appropriate.

- Utilizes the plan of care to provide direction and regular updates to other members of the healthcare team.

- Defines the plan of care to reflect current statutes, rules and regulations, and standards.

- Integrates current best practices and research affecting care in the planning process.

- Considers the economic impact of the plan of care.

- Uses standardized language or recognized terminology to document the plan of care.

- Communicates to other interdisciplinary team members and consultants.

Additional Measurement Criteria for the Advanced Practice Hospice and Palliative Registered Nurse:

The advanced practice hospice and palliative registered nurse:

- Identifies assessment, diagnostic strategies, and therapeutic interventions within the plan of care that reflect current evidence, including data, research, literature, expert clinical knowledge, and collaboration from others when necessary.

- Selects or designs strategies to meet the multifaceted needs of complex patients, and physiological and psychosocial changes common to all ages, including consulting with other experts in developing the plan of care.

- Includes the synthesis of patient and family values and beliefs regarding nursing and medical therapies within the plan of care.

Additional Measurement Criteria for the Hospice and Palliative Registered Nurse in a Nursing Role Specialty:

The hospice and palliative registered nurse in a nursing role specialty:

- Participates in the design and development of multidisciplinary and interdisciplinary processes to address the typical life-limiting, progressive illness.

- Contributes to the development and continuous improvement of organizational systems that support the planning process.

- Supports the integration of clinical, human, and financial resources to enhance and complete the critical thinking needed in planning processes.

STANDARD 5. IMPLEMENTATION
The hospice and palliative registered nurse implements the identified plan of care.

Measurement Criteria:

The hospice and palliative registered nurse:

- Implements the plan of care in a safe, timely, and culturally competent manner.

- Documents implementation and any modifications, including changes or omissions, of the identified plan of care.

- Utilizes evidence-based interventions and treatments specific to the diagnoses or problems.

- Collaborates with patient, family members, nursing colleagues, interdisciplinary team, and others to implement the plan of care.

- Utilizes community resources and systems to implement the plan of care.

- Promotes quality of life for individuals and families by relieving suffering.

- Advocates to promote self-determination, resolve conflicts, and ensure ethically appropriate care.

Additional Measurement Criteria for the Advanced Practice Hospice and Palliative Registered Nurse:

The advanced practice hospice and palliative registered nurse:

- Facilitates identification and utilization of systems and community resources to implement the plan.

- Collaborates with patients, family members, nursing colleagues, the palliative care interdisciplinary team, and other appropriate healthcare providers to implement the plan.

- Incorporates new knowledge and strategies to initiate change in nursing care practices if desired outcomes are not achieved.

Additional Measurement Criteria for the Hospice and Palliative Registered Nurse in a Nursing Role Specialty:

The hospice and palliative registered nurse in a nursing role specialty:

- Implements the plan using principles and concepts of project or systems management.

- Fosters organizational systems that support implementation of the plan of care.

STANDARD 5A: COORDINATION OF CARE
The hospice and palliative registered nurse coordinates care delivery.

Measurement Criteria:

The hospice and palliative registered nurse:

- Coordinates implementation of the plan of care.

- Documents the coordination of interdisciplinary care.

- Considers the complexity of coordination of care for patients of all ages, their families, and caregivers.

Measurement Criteria for the Advanced Practice Hospice and Palliative Registered Nurse:

The advanced practice hospice and palliative registered nurse:

- Provides leadership in the coordination of interdisciplinary health care for integrated delivery of patient care services.

- Synthesizes data and information to prescribe necessary medications, treatments, consultations, and system and community support measures, including environmental modifications.

- Coordinates system and community resources that enhance delivery of care across the healthcare continuum.

STANDARD 5B: HEALTH TEACHING AND HEALTH PROMOTION
The hospice and palliative registered nurse employs strategies to promote health and a safe environment.

Measurement Criteria:

The hospice and palliative registered nurse:

- Provides health teaching that addresses such topics as healthy lifestyles, risk-reducing behaviors, developmental needs, activities of daily living, and preventive self-care.

- Uses health promotion and health teaching methods appropriate to the situation and the patient's developmental level, learning needs, readiness, ability to learn, language preference, spiritual preference, and culture.

- Seeks opportunities for feedback and evaluation of the effectiveness of the strategies used.

Additional Measurement Criteria for the Advanced Practice Hospice and Palliative Registered Nurse:

The advanced practice hospice and palliative registered nurse:

- Synthesizes empirical evidence on risk behaviors, learning theories, behavioral change theories, motivational theories, epidemiology, and other related theories and frameworks when designing health information and patient and family education.

- Designs health information and education for the patient and family appropriate to their developmental level, learning needs, readiness to learn, and cultural values and beliefs.

- Utilizes geriatric best practices as a basis for health promotion, maintenance, and teaching related to older adults, their families, and caregivers.

- Evaluates health information resources, including the Internet, within the area of practice for accuracy, readability, and comprehensibility to help patients access quality health information.

STANDARD 5C: CONSULTATION

The advanced practice hospice and palliative registered nurse and the nursing role specialist provide consultation to influence the identified plan, enhance the abilities of others, and effect change.

Measurement Criteria for the Advanced Practice Hospice and Palliative Registered Nurse:

The advanced hospice and palliative practice registered nurse:

- Synthesizes clinical data, theoretical frameworks, and evidence when providing consultation.
- Facilitates the effectiveness of a consultation by involving the patient and family in decision making and negotiating role responsibilities.
- Communicates consultation recommendations that facilitate change for the patient, family, and all caregivers.

Measurement Criteria for the Hospice and Palliative Registered Nurse in a Nursing Role Specialty:

The hospice and palliative registered nurse in a nursing role specialty:

- Synthesizes data, information, theoretical frameworks, and evidence when providing consultation.
- Facilitates the effectiveness of a consultation by involving the stakeholders in the decision-making process.
- Communicates consultation recommendations that influence the identified plan.
- Facilitates understanding by involved stakeholders, enhancing the work of others and effecting change.

STANDARD 5D: PRESCRIPTIVE AUTHORITY AND TREATMENT

The advanced practice hospice and palliative registered nurse uses prescriptive authority, procedures, referrals, treatments, and therapies in accordance with state and federal laws and regulations.

Measurement Criteria for the Advanced Practice Hospice and Palliative Registered Nurse:

The advanced practice hospice and palliative registered nurse:

- Prescribes evidence-based treatments, therapies, and procedures considering the patient's comprehensive healthcare needs.

- Prescribes pharmacologic agents based on a current knowledge of pharmacology, physiology and physiologic changes, pharmacodynamic, and medication adherence common to older adults.

- Prescribes specific pharmacological agents and treatments based on clinical indicators, the patient's status and needs, and the results of diagnostic and laboratory tests.

- Orders referral or consults to other disciplines to meet the patient's needs (e.g., physical therapy, behavioral medicine, massage therapy, healing touch).

- Evaluates therapeutic and potential adverse effects of pharmacological and non-pharmacological treatments.

- Provides patients with information about intended effects and potential adverse effects of proposed prescriptive therapies.

- Provides information about financial considerations of evidence-based therapies, and alternative treatments and procedures, as appropriate.

STANDARD 6. EVALUATION
The hospice and palliative registered nurse evaluates progress towards attainment of outcomes.

Measurement Criteria:

The hospice and palliative registered nurse:

- Conducts a systematic, ongoing, and criterion-based evaluation of the outcomes in relation to the structures and processes prescribed by the plan of care and the indicated timeline.
- Includes the patient, family, and others involved in the care or situation in the evaluative process.
- Evaluates the effectiveness of the planned strategies in relation to patient responses and the attainment of the expected outcomes.
- Documents the results of the evaluation.
- Uses ongoing assessment data to revise the nursing diagnoses, outcomes, the plan of care, and the implementation as needed.
- Disseminates the evaluation results to the patient, family, interdisciplinary team, and others involved in the care or situation, as appropriate, in accordance with state and federal laws and regulations.

Additional Measurement Criteria for the Advanced Practice Hospice and Palliative Registered Nurse:

The advanced practice hospice and palliative registered nurse:

- Evaluates the accuracy of the diagnosis and effectiveness of the interventions in relationship to the patient's attainment of expected outcomes.
- Synthesizes the results of the evaluation analyses to determine the impact of the plan of care on the affected patients, families, groups, communities, and institutions.
- Uses the results of the evaluation analyses to make or recommend process or structural changes including policy, procedure, or protocol documentation, as appropriate.

Additional Measurement Criteria for the Hospice and Palliative Registered Nurse in a Nursing Role Specialty:

The hospice and palliative registered nurse in a nursing role specialty:

- Uses the results of the evaluation analyses to make or recommend process or structural changes including policy, procedure, or protocol documentation, as appropriate.

- Synthesizes the results of the evaluation analyses to determine the impact of the plan on the affected patients, families, groups, communities, institutions, networks, and organizations.

STANDARDS OF PROFESSIONAL PERFORMANCE

STANDARD 7. QUALITY OF PRACTICE
The hospice and palliative registered nurse systematically enhances the quality and effectiveness of nursing practice.

Measurement Criteria:

The hospice and palliative registered nurse:

- Demonstrates quality by documenting the application of the nursing process in a responsible, accountable, and ethical manner.

- Uses the results of quality improvement activities to initiate changes in nursing practice and in the healthcare delivery system.

- Uses creativity and innovation in nursing practice to improve care delivery.

- Incorporates new knowledge to initiate changes in nursing practice if desired outcomes are not achieved.

- Participates in quality improvement activities. Such activities may include:

    - Identifying aspects of practice important for quality monitoring.

    - Using indicators developed to monitor quality and effectiveness of nursing practice.

    - Collecting data to monitor quality and effectiveness of nursing practice.

    - Analyzing quality data to identify opportunities for improving nursing practice.

    - Formulating recommendations to improve nursing practice or outcomes.

    - Implementing activities to enhance the quality of nursing practice.

    - Developing, implementing, and evaluating policies, procedures, and guidelines to improve the quality of practice.

Continued ▶

- Participating on interdisciplinary teams to evaluate clinical care or health services.
- Participating in efforts to minimize costs and unnecessary duplication.
- Analyzing factors related to safety, satisfaction, effectiveness, and cost–benefit options.
- Analyzing organizational systems for barriers.
- Implementing processes to remove or decrease barriers within organizational systems.

Additional Measurement Criteria for the Advanced Practice Hospice and Palliative Registered Nurse:

The advanced practice hospice and palliative registered nurse:

- Obtains and maintains professional certification in the area of expertise.
- Designs quality improvement initiatives.
- Implements initiatives to evaluate the need for change within organizational systems.
- Evaluates the practice environment and quality of nursing care rendered in relation to existing evidence, identifying opportunities for the generation and use of research.
- Bases evaluation on current knowledge, practice, and research common to older adults.
- Participates in research activities.

Additional Measurement Criteria for the Hospice and Palliative Registered Nurse in a Nursing Role Specialty:

The hospice and palliative registered nurse in a nursing role specialty:

- Obtains and maintains professional certification if available in the area of expertise.
- Designs quality improvement initiatives.
- Implements initiatives to evaluate the need for change.
- Evaluates the practice environment in relation to existing evidence, identifying opportunities for the generation and use of research.

STANDARD 8. EDUCATION
The hospice and palliative registered nurse attains knowledge and competency that reflects current hospice and palliative nursing practice.

Measurement Criteria:

The hospice and palliative registered nurse:

- Participates in ongoing educational activities related to appropriate knowledge bases and professional issues.

- Demonstrates a commitment to lifelong learning through self-reflection and inquiry to identify learning needs.

- Seeks experiences that reflect current practice in order to maintain skills and competence in clinical practice or role performance.

- Acquires knowledge and skills appropriate to the specialty area, practice setting, role, or situation.

- Maintains professional records that provide evidence of competency and life long learning.

- Seeks experiences and formal and independent learning activities to maintain and develop clinical and professional skills and knowledge.

Additional Measurement Criteria for the Advanced Practice Hospice and Palliative Registered Nurse:

The advanced practice hospice and palliative registered nurse:

- Uses current healthcare research findings and other evidence to expand clinical knowledge, enhance role performance, and increase knowledge of professional issues.

- Provides inservice education to others in the area of interest.

- Provides presentations to local, state, national, and international conferences in area of expertise.

- Offers to precept nursing and other professional students.

- Educates advocates, lobbyists, and politicians as needed on nursing and healthcare issues.

Continued ▶

Additional Measurement Criteria for the Hospice and Palliative Registered Nurse in a Nursing Role Specialty:

The hospice and palliative registered nurse in a nursing role specialty:

- Uses current research findings and other evidence to expand knowledge, enhance role performance, and increase knowledge of professional issues.
- Precepts nursing students, new employees, and ancillary staff.

STANDARD 9. PROFESSIONAL PRACTICE EVALUATION

The hospice and palliative registered nurse evaluates one's own nursing practice in relation to professional practice standards and guidelines, relevant statutes, rules, and regulations.

Measurement Criteria:

The hospice and palliative registered nurse's practice reflects the application of knowledge of current practice standards, guidelines, statutes, rules, and regulations.

The hospice and palliative registered nurse:

- Provides age-appropriate care in a culturally and ethnically sensitive manner.

- Engages in self-evaluation of practice on a regular basis, identifying areas of strength as well as areas in which professional development would be beneficial.

- Obtains informal feedback regarding one's own practice from patients, peers, professional colleagues, and others.

- Participates in systematic peer review as appropriate.

- Takes action to achieve goals identified during the evaluation process.

- Provides rationales for practice beliefs, decisions, and actions as part of the informal and formal evaluation processes.

Additional Measurement Criteria for the Advanced Practice Hospice and Palliative Registered Nurse:

The advanced practice hospice and palliative registered nurse:

- Engages in a peer review formal process seeking feedback regarding one's own practice from patients, peers, professional colleagues, and others.

- Provides constructive and sensitive feedback to others regarding their practice with a focus on improvement of nursing practice and achievement of excellence.

Continued ▶

Additional Measurement Criteria for the Hospice and Palliative Registered Nurse in a Nursing Role Specialty:

The hospice and palliative registered nurse in a nursing role specialty:

- Engages in a formal process seeking feedback regarding role performance from individuals, professional colleagues, representatives and administrators of corporate entities, and others.

STANDARD 10. COLLEGIALITY

The hospice and palliative registered nurse interacts with and contributes to the professional development of peers and colleagues.

Measurement Criteria:

The hospice and palliative registered nurse:

- Shares knowledge and skills with peers and colleagues as evidenced by such activities as patient care conferences or presentations at formal or informal meetings.
- Provides peers with feedback regarding their practice and role performance.
- Interacts with peers and colleagues to enhance one's own professional nursing practice and role performance.
- Maintains compassionate and caring relationships with peers and colleagues.
- Contributes to an environment that is conducive to the education of healthcare professionals.
- Contributes to a supportive and healthy work environment.

Additional Measurement Criteria for the Advanced Practice Hospice and Palliative Registered Nurse:

The advanced practice hospice and palliative registered nurse:

- Models expert practice to interdisciplinary team members and healthcare consumers.
- Mentors other registered nurses and colleagues as appropriate.
- Participates with interdisciplinary teams that contribute to role development and advanced nursing practice and health care.
- Assesses the emotional climate of the work environment and takes appropriate actions to improve the situation.
- Assesses the emotional, spiritual, and social needs of others on the interdisciplinary team and takes appropriate action to assist those in distress.

Continued ▶

Additional Measurement Criteria for the Hospice and Palliative Registered Nurse in a Nursing Role Specialty:

The hospice and palliative registered nurse in a nursing role specialty:

- Participates on interdisciplinary and multi-professional teams that contribute to role development and, directly or indirectly, advance nursing practice and health services.

- Mentors other hospice and palliative registered nurses and colleagues as appropriate.

- Assists new interdisciplinary team members to become part of the team.

STANDARD 11. COLLABORATION

The hospice and palliative registered nurse collaborates with the patient, the family, the interdisciplinary team, and others in the conduct of nursing practice.

Measurement Criteria:

The hospice and palliative registered nurse:

- Communicates with the patient, the family, the interdisciplinary team, and healthcare providers regarding patient care and the nurse's role in the provision of that care.

- Collaborates in creating a documented plan focused on outcomes and decisions related to care and delivery of services that indicates communication with patients, families, and others.

- Partners with others to effect change and generate positive outcomes through knowledge of the patient, family, or situation.

- Documents referrals, including provisions for continuity of care.

Additional Measurement Criteria for the Advanced Practice Hospice and Palliative Registered Nurse:

The advanced practice hospice and palliative registered nurse:

- Partners with other disciplines to enhance patient care through interdisciplinary activities such as education, consultation, management, technological development, or research opportunities.

- Facilitates an interdisciplinary process with other members of the healthcare team.

- Documents plan-of-care communications, rationales for plan-of-care changes, and collaborative discussions to improve patient care.

Continued ▶

Additional Measurement Criteria for the Hospice and Palliative Registered Nurse in a Nursing Role Specialty:

The hospice and palliative registered nurse in a nursing role specialty:

- Partners with others to enhance health care and ultimately patient care, through interdisciplinary activities such as education, consultation, management, technological development, or research opportunities.

- Participates in the revision process of local, state, and federal regulations when possible.

- Documents plans, communications, rationales for plan-of-care changes and collaborative discussions with consideration of regulatory and governmental constraints.

STANDARD 12. ETHICS

The hospice and palliative registered nurse integrates ethical provisions in all areas of practice.

Measurement Criteria:

The hospice and palliative registered nurse:

- Uses *Code of Ethics for Nurses with Interpretive Statements* (ANA, 2001) to guide practice.

- Delivers care in a manner that preserves and protects patient autonomy, cultural preferences, dignity, and rights, and honors the patient's wishes.

- Maintains patient confidentiality within legal and regulatory parameters.

- Actively participates in the informed consent process (including the right to choose) for patients' procedures, tests, treatments, and research participation, as appropriate, by educating, advocating, and clarifying options to the patient and family.

- Serves as a patient advocate, assisting patients in developing skills for self advocacy.

- Maintains a therapeutic and professional patient–nurse relationship within appropriate professional role boundaries.

- Demonstrates a commitment to practicing self-care, managing stress, and connecting with self and others.

- Contributes to resolving ethical issues of patients, colleagues, or systems as evidenced in such activities as requesting an ethics consult in a confidential, non-punitive manner.

- Reports illegal, incompetent, or impaired practices.

Continued ▶

Additional Measurement Criteria for the Advanced Practice Hospice and Palliative Registered Nurse:

The advanced practice hospice and palliative registered nurse:

- Informs the patient of the risks, benefits, and outcomes of health-care regimens.

- Participates in interdisciplinary teams that address ethical risks, benefits, and outcomes of practice.

- Articulates a working knowledge of end-of-life ethical issues, including state law regarding Do Not Resuscitate, research pros and cons of artificial nutrition, state law on ethical concerns regarding withdrawal of life support, etc.

Additional Measurement Criteria for the Hospice and Palliative Registered Nurse in a Nursing Role Specialty:

The hospice and palliative registered nurse in a nursing role specialty:

- Participates on multidisciplinary and interdisciplinary teams that address ethical risks, benefits, and outcomes.

- Informs administrators or others of the risks, benefits, and outcomes of programs and decisions that affect healthcare delivery.

Standard 13. Research
The hospice and palliative registered nurse integrates research findings into practice.

Measurement Criteria:

The hospice and palliative registered nurse:

- Utilizes the best available evidence, including research findings, to guide practice decisions.

- Actively participates in research activities at various levels appropriate to the nurse's level of education and position. Such activities may include:

  - Identifying clinical problems specific to nursing research (patient care and nursing practice).

  - Participating in data collection (surveys, pilot projects, formal studies).

  - Participating in a formal committee or program.

  - Sharing research activities and findings with peers and others.

  - Conducting research.

  - Critically analyzing and interpreting research for application to practice.

  - Using research findings in the development of policies, procedures, and standards of practice in patient care.

  - Incorporating research as a basis for learning methods to improve patient care.

Additional Measurement Criteria for the Advanced Practice Hospice and Palliative Registered Nurse:

The advanced practice hospice and palliative registered nurse:

- Contributes to nursing knowledge by conducting or synthesizing research that discovers, examines, and evaluates knowledge, theories, criteria, and creative approaches to improve healthcare practice.

- Formally disseminates research findings through activities such as presentations, publications, consultation, and journal clubs.

Continued ▶

Additional Measurement Criteria for the Hospice and Palliative Registered Nurse in a Nursing Role Specialty:

The hospice and palliative registered nurse in a nursing role specialty:

- Contributes to nursing knowledge by conducting or synthesizing research that discovers, examines, and evaluates knowledge, theories, criteria, and creative approaches to improve health care within the required regulations.

- Formally disseminates research findings through activities such as presentations, publications, consultation, and journal clubs.

STANDARD 14. RESOURCE UTILIZATION

The hospice and palliative registered nurse considers factors related to safety, effectiveness, cost, and impact on practice in the planning and delivery of nursing services.

Measurement Criteria:

The hospice and palliative registered nurse:

- Evaluates factors such as safety, effectiveness, availability, cost and benefits, efficiencies, and impact on practice, when choosing practice options that would result in the same expected outcome.

- Assists the patient and family in identifying and securing appropriate and available services to address health-related needs.

- Assigns or delegates tasks, based on the needs and condition of the patient, potential for harm, stability of the patient's condition, complexity of the task, and predictability of the outcome.

- Assists the patient and family in becoming informed consumers about the options, costs, risks, and benefits of treatment and care.

Additional Measurement Criteria for the Advanced Practice Hospice and Palliative Registered Nurse:

The advanced practice hospice and palliative registered nurse:

- Utilizes organizational and community resources to formulate multidisciplinary or interdisciplinary plans of care.

- Develops innovative solutions for patient care problems that address effective resource utilization and maintenance of quality.

- Develops evaluation strategies to demonstrate cost effectiveness, cost benefit, and efficiency factors associated with nursing practice.

Continued ▶

Additional Measurement Criteria for the Hospice and Palliative Registered Nurse in a Nursing Role Specialty:

The hospice and palliative registered nurse in a nursing role specialty:

- Develops innovative solutions and applies strategies to obtain appropriate resources for nursing initiatives.

- Secures organizational resources to ensure a work environment conducive to completing the identified plan and outcomes.

- Develops evaluation methods to measure safety and effectiveness for interventions and outcomes.

- Promotes activities that assist others, as appropriate, in becoming informed about costs, risks, and benefits of care or of the plan and solution.

STANDARD 15. LEADERSHIP
The hospice and palliative registered nurse provides leadership in the professional practice setting and the profession.

Measurement Criteria:

The hospice and palliative registered nurse:

- Engages in teamwork as a team player, a team builder, and a team leader.

- Works to create and maintain healthy work environments.

- Displays the ability to define a clear vision of associated goals and to plan, implement, and measure progress.

- Demonstrates a commitment to continuous, lifelong learning for self and others.

- Facilitates teaching others to succeed by mentoring and other strategies.

- Exhibits creativity and flexibility through times of change.

- Demonstrates energy, excitement, joy, and a passion for quality work.

- Willingly accepts mistakes by self and others, thereby creating a culture in which risk-taking is not only safe but expected.

- Inspires loyalty through valuing of people as the most precious asset in an organization.

- Directs the coordination of care across settings and among caregivers, including oversight of licensed and unlicensed personnel in any assigned or delegated tasks.

- Serves in key roles in the work setting by participating on committees, councils, and administrative teams.

- Promotes advancement of the profession through participation in professional organizations.

Continued ▶

Additional Measurement Criteria for the Advanced Practice Hospice and Palliative Registered Nurse:

The advanced practice hospice and palliative registered nurse:

- Works to influence decision-making bodies to improve patient care.

- Provides direction to enhance the effectiveness of the healthcare team.

- Initiates and revises protocols or guidelines to reflect evidence-based or best practices, to reflect accepted changes in care management, or to address emerging problems.

- Promotes communication of information and advancement of the profession through writing, publishing, and presentations for professional or lay audiences.

- Designs innovations to effect change in practice and improve health outcomes.

Additional Measurement Criteria for the Hospice and Palliative Registered Nurse in a Nursing Role Specialty:

The hospice and palliative registered nurse in a nursing role specialty:

- Works to influence decision-making bodies to improve patient care, health services, and policies.

- Promotes communication of information and advancement of the profession through writing, publishing, and presentations for professional or lay audiences.

- Designs innovations to effect change in practice and outcomes.

- Provides direction to enhance the effectiveness of the multi-disciplinary or interdisciplinary team.

Glossary

Admission process. The activity that begins with the initial referral to the program of care and continues through the development of the interdisciplinary plan of care.

Assessment. A systematic, dynamic process in which the nurse, through interaction with the patient and family, significant others, other members of the interdisciplinary healthcare team, and consultants, collects and analyzes data about the patient and family. Data may include physical, psychological, sociocultural, spiritual, cognitive, functional, developmental, economic, and lifestyle dimensions.

Continuity of care. An interdisciplinary process that includes patients and significant others in the development of a coordinated plan of care. This process facilitates the patient's transition between settings, based on changing needs and available resources, across the healthcare continuum.

Criteria. Relevant, measurable indicators of the standards of hospice and palliative nursing practice.

Diagnosis. The analysis and synthesis of the patient history, physical examination, and test results to formulate a hypothesis of an abnormal condition indicated by the anatomy, physiology, or biochemical dysfunction of an organ.

Evaluation. The process of determining both the patient's and the family's progress toward the attainment of expected outcomes and the effectiveness of nursing care, including the patient's value system and goals for care.

Family. People bound by biological or legal ties, or those who define themselves as a "close other" with another person, or "those who function in familistic ways" (Settles, 1987, p. 160). These ways of functioning can include nurturance, intimacy, companionship, and economic, social, psychosocial, spiritual, and physical support in time of need or in illness (adapted from Matocha, 1992).

Healthcare providers. People with special expertise who provide healthcare services or assistance to patients. They must include nurses, physicians, pharmacists, patient care technicians, psychologists, social workers, nutritionists/dietitians, various therapists (such as physical therapists, occupational therapists, and speech and language therapists), and other members of the interdisciplinary team, such as chaplains or spiritual counselors.

Implementation. Any of the following activities: teaching, intervening, delegating, and coordinating. The patient and family or other members of the interdisciplinary healthcare team may be designated to implement interventions in the plan of care.

Interdisciplinary team. A highly qualified, specially trained team of hospice and palliative care professionals and volunteers who work together to meet the physiological, psychological, social, spiritual, and economic needs of the patient and family facing life-limiting, progressive illness and bereavement. The team may include physicians, nurses, social workers, clergy, bereavement counselors, and others as indicated for specific needs.

Life-limiting illness. Any chronic illness that is life threatening and progressively debilitating regardless of age, length of time since diagnosis or functional status.

Nurse. A person licensed by a state agency to practice as a registered nurse.

Nursing. The protection, promotion, and optimization of health and abilities, prevention of illness and injury, alleviation of suffering through the diagnosis and treatment of human response, and advocacy in the care of individuals, families, communities, and populations (ANA, 2003, p. 6).

Nursing diagnoses. A clinical judgment about the patient's and family's response to actual or potential health conditions or needs. Nursing diagnoses most often focus on pain and symptom management and provide the basis for determination of a plan of care to achieve expected outcomes.

Nursing role specialty. An advanced level of nursing practice that intersects with another body of knowledge, has a direct influence on nursing practice, and supports the delivery of direct care rendered to patients by other professional nurses (ANA, 2004, p. 16).

Outcomes. Measurable expected patient- and family-focused goals that translate into observable behaviors.

Palliative care continuum. Support and care for people and their families experiencing life-limiting, progressive illness from the time of diagnosis with advanced disease or serious injury through the death of the person and into the bereavement period of the family.

Patient. Recipient of nursing practice. The term *patient* is used in the standards to provide consistency and brevity, bearing in mind that *client* or *individual* might be better choices in some instances. When the patient is one person, the focus is on the health, problems, or needs of that person. When the patient is a family or group, the focus is on the health state of the unit as a whole or the effects of an individual's health on the other members of the unit.

Plan of care. The comprehensive outline of care, written according to the patient's or family's wishes and intended to attain expected outcomes when implemented by the interdisciplinary team.

Resources. Assets that can be drawn upon by the patient and family for aid. Types of resources include, but are not limited to, financial, emotional, spiritual, social, psychological, and physical.

Standard. An authoritative statement enunciated and promulgated by the profession, by which the quality of practice, service, or education can be judged.

Standards of practice. Authoritative statements that describe a competent level of nursing care as demonstrated by the critical thinking model known as the nursing process. The nursing process includes assessment, diagnosis, outcomes identification, planning, implementation, and evaluation. The nursing process encompasses all significant actions taken by registered nurses, and is the foundation of the nurse's decision making (ANA, 2004, p. 4).

Standards of professional performance. Authoritative statements that describe a competent level of behavior in the professional role, including activities related to quality of practice, education, professional practice evaluation, collegiality, collaboration, ethics, research, resource utilization, and leadership (ANA, 2004, p. 4).

Unit of care. The patient with a life-limiting or progressive illness and the patient's family. The patient and family are an interdependent, integrated whole composed of two or more individuals. They experience individual as well as overlapping needs.

REFERENCES

American Association of Colleges of Nursing (AACN). (1997). *Peaceful death document*. Washington, DC: AACN.

American Association of Colleges of Nursing (AACN) and City of Hope National Medical Center. (2005). *End-of-Life Nursing Education Consortium (ELNEC) Project*.

American Nurses Association (ANA). (2001). *Code of ethics for nurses with interpretive statements*. Washington, DC: American Nurses Publishing.

American Nurses Association (ANA). (2003). *Pain management and control of distressing symptoms in dying patients*. Available under Position Statements: Ethics and Human Rights at http://www.nursingworld.org.

Center to Advance Palliative Care (CAPC). (2006). Hospital Palliative Care Programs Continue Rapid Growth. (December 7, 2006). CAPC, New York, NY. Available at http://www.capc.org/news-and-events/releases/december-2006-release.

Hospice and Palliative Nurses Association (HPNA). (2001). *Professional competencies for generalist hospice and palliative nurses*. Dubuque, IA: Kendall/Hunt.

Hospice and Palliative Nurses Association (HPNA). (2002). *Competencies for advance practice hospice and palliative care nurses*. Dubuque, IA: Kendall/Hunt.

Knaus, W. et al. (1995). A controlled trial to improve care for seriously ill hospitalized patients. *Journal of the American Medical Association 274* (20), 1591–1598.

Last Acts Task Force. (1998). National policy statements on end-of-life care: Precepts of palliative care. *Journal of Palliative Medicine 1,* 109–112.

Matocha, L. K. (1992). Case study interviews: Caring for persons with AIDS. In J. F. Gilgun, K. Daly, & G. Handel (Eds.), *Qualitative methods in family research* (pp. 66–84). Newbury Park, CA: Sage Publications.

National Consensus Project for Quality Palliative Care. (2004). *Clinical practice guidelines for quality palliative care.* http://www.nationalconsensusproject.org.

Settles, B. H. (1987). A perspective on tomorrow's families. In M. B. Sussman & S. K. Steinmetz (Eds.), *Handbook of marriage and the family* (pp. 157–180). New York: Plenum.

BIBLIOGRAPHY

Billings, J. A., & Block, S. (1997). Palliative care in undergraduate medical education. *Journal of the American Medical Association 278* (9), 733–736.

Dahlin, C. (1999). Access to Hospice. In I. Corless & Z. Foster (Eds.), *The Hospice Heritage: Celebrating the future* (pp. 75–84). New York: The Haworth Press, Inc.

Doyle, D., Hanks, G., & MacDonald, N. (1998). *Oxford textbook of palliative medicine.* New York: Oxford Medical Publication.

Ferris, F., & Cummings, I. (1995). *Palliative care: Towards a consensus in standardized principles of practice.* Ottawa, Ontario: Canadian Palliative Care Association.

Field, M., & Cassel, C. (1997). *Approaching death: Improving care at the end of life.* Washington, DC: National Academy Press.

Portenoy, R., & Bruera, B. (1997). *Topics in palliative care: Volume 1.* New York: Oxford Medical Publications.

Randall, F., & Downie, R. S. (1996). *Palliative care ethics.* New York: Oxford Medical Publications.

Sherman, D. W. (2001). Access to hospice care. *Journal of Palliative Medicine, 3*(4), 407–411.

APPENDIX A.
SCOPE AND STANDARDS OF HOSPICE AND PALLIATIVE NURSING PRACTICE (2002)

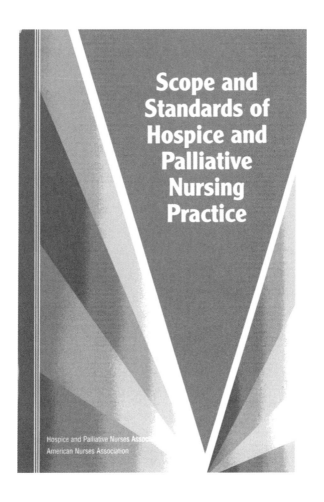

Scope and Standards of Hospice and Palliative Nursing Practice

Hospice and Palliative Nurses Association

American Nurses Association

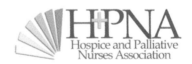

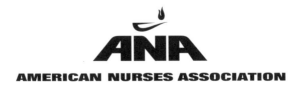

Washington, D.C.

Library of Congress Cataloging-in-Publication Data

Hospice and Palliative Nurses Association.
Scope and standards of hospice and palliative nursing practice / Hospice
and Palliative Nurses Association, American Nurses Association.
    p. ; cm.
Includes bibliographical references.
  ISBN 1-55810-207-8 (alk. paper)
  1. Hospice care. 2. Nursing. 3. Palliative treatment.
  [DNLM: 1. Hospice Care—standards—United States. 2. Nursing Care—
standards—United States. 3. Palliative Care—standards—United States.
WB 310 H8283 2002]
  I. American Nurses Association.
  II. Title.
  R726.8 H6533 2002
  610.73'61—dc21

                                                          2002152410

Development of these Standards was made possible in part by a grant from
New York University and Project Death in America.

Published by
American Nurses Publishing
600 Maryland Avenue, SW
Suite 100 West
Washington, D.C. 20024-2571

ISBN 1-55810-207-8

HPN22   2M   11/02

Authors
Patsy Abbott, RN, BSN, CHPN
Susan Derby, RN, MA, CGNP
Constance Dahlin, MSN, RNCS, CRNH
Michael Ryan, MSN, BSN, CRNH
Denice Sheehan, MSN, RN
Deborah Sherman, PhD, RN, ANP, CS

Reviewers
Clare Conner, MSN, BSN, RN
Pamela Fordham, RN, DSN, FNP-C
Linda Gorman, MN, RN, CHPN

Editors
Constance Dahlin, MSN, RNCS, CRNH
Judy Lentz, RN, MSN, OCN, NHA

Office of Nursing Policy and Practice, American Nurses Association
Carol Bickford, PhD, RN
Yvonne Humes

Contents

PREFACE

This document was developed by the Hospice and Palliative Nurses Education Committee Task Force on Scope and Standards. This is the third edition. The first edition focused on basic hospice nursing. The second edition brought together the aspects of both hospice and palliative care. This third edition of the Statement on the Scope and Standards, written by the organization, advances practice forward yet again by addressing both generalist and advanced practice hospice and palliative nursing.

The Hospice and Palliative Nurses Association Education/Research Committee acknowledges the work of the Advanced Practice Competency Task Force for their initial work on this project supported by funds from a grant from New York University (NYU) and Project Death in America. This task force, led by Deborah Sherman, was a result of collaborative efforts from NYU and the National Board for Certification of Hospice and Palliative Nursing to develop an advanced practice nursing certification process. The APN Task Force built on the foundational work of the Generalist Nurse Competency Task Force to begin comparing and contrasting the work of generalist and advanced practice nurses. This work was further developed and approved by the Hospice and Palliative Nurses Association. We are fortunate to have benefited from a collective wealth of knowledge and experience.

It is our hope that this helps to further develop the practice of hospice and palliative care and to set standards for all registered nurses and advanced practice nurses who practice within the realm of end of life care.

INTRODUCTION

By developing and articulating the scope and standards of professional nursing practice, the specialty of hospice and palliative nursing informs society about the parameters of nursing practice and guides states in the development of rules and regulations determining hospice and palliative nursing practice. However, because each state creates its own laws and regulations governing nursing, the designated limits, function, and titles for nurses, especially those for advanced practice, may vary significantly from state to state. As in all nursing specialties, hospice and palliative nurses must accept professional practice accountability and ensure that their practice remains within the scope of their state nurse practice act, professional code of ethics, and professional practice standards. The first Standards of Hospice nursing practice were developed in 1987 for the American Nurses Association and were revised in 1995. This revision of the 2000 *Statement of the Scope and Standards of Hospice and Palliative Nursing Practice* incorporates the advanced level of nursing practice.

Nursing practice is differentiated according to the nurse's educational preparation and level of practice. The hospice and palliative care nurse may practice from a generalist through advanced level of competency. In this document, the title Advanced Practice Nurse (APN) is used as an inclusive term to describe the common core of knowledge, skills, and abilities of both the Clinical Nurse Specialist (CNS) and the Nurse Practitioner (NP). In many practice settings, a blended role exists that combines the strengths of the CNS and NP, while the differences between the two are based on the focus of service. The blended role of the advanced practice hospice and palliative nurse demonstrates advanced competencies to promote the quality of life for individuals and their families experiencing life-limiting, progressive illness.

Evolutionary Perspective of Hospice and Palliative Nursing

The landmark SUPPORT study (Study to Understand Prognoses and Preferences for Outcomes and Risk of Treatment) by Knaus et al. (1995) highlights an urgent need for healthcare professionals who are prepared and committed to improving the quality of life for seriously ill and dying patients and their families. Knaus et al. (1995) conducted a 2-year prospective observational study with 4,301 patients from teaching hospitals in the United States, followed by a 2-year controlled clinical trial with 4,804 patients and their physicians who were either randomized to a control group or to an intervention group that received educational information related to the end of life. The findings indicated that, despite the SUPPORT intervention, there was:

- A continued lack of communication between patients and their providers, particularly related to end-of-life preferences;
- An aggressiveness of medical treatments; and
- A high level of reported pain by seriously ill and dying patients.

Knaus et al. (1995) believe that improving the experience of seriously ill and dying patients requires an individual and collective commitment of healthcare providers as well as proactive efforts at shaping the caregiving process. Having invested 28 million dollars in the SUPPORT study, the Robert Wood Johnson Foundation (RWJF) has extended its commitment to end-of-life care, recognizing the "overriding need to change the kind of care dying Americans receive" (Last Acts Task Force, 1998).

It has been recognized that educational preparation for end-of-life care is inconsistent at best, and neglected for the most part, in both undergraduate and graduate curricula (AACN, 1997). In accord with the International Council of Nurses' mandate that nurses have a unique and primary responsibility for ensuring the peaceful death of patients, the American Association of Colleges of Nursing, supported by the Robert Wood Johnson Foundation, convened a round table of expert nurses to discuss and initiate educational change related to palliative care. It was concluded that precepts underlying hospice care are essential principles for all end-of-life care. Such precepts include the assumptions that:

- Persons are living until the moment of death;
- Coordinated care should be offered by a variety of professionals with attention to the physical, psychological, social, and spiritual needs of patients and their families; and
- Care be sensitive to patient/family diversity.

It was proposed that these precepts be foundational content in the educational preparation of nurses. Based on these precepts, the document "Peaceful Death" was developed, which outlined baccalaureate competencies for palliative/hospice care and the content areas where these competencies can be taught (AACN, 1997).

Emphasizing the role of nursing in end-of-life care, the American Nurses Association formulated a position statement regarding the promotion of comfort and relief of pain of dying patients, reinforcing the nurse's obligation to promote comfort and ensure aggressive efforts to relieve pain and suffering. Initiatives are underway in nursing to include palliative care content in licensing examinations and to revise nursing textbooks to include palliative care content. Specialized palliative care educational initiatives have also begun, such as the End of Life Nursing Education Consortium, (ELNEC), supported by a major grant from the Robert Wood Johnson Foundation to the American Association of Colleges of Nursing and City of Hope Medical Center. One goal of ELNEC is to train 1,000 nurse educators from associate degree and baccalaureate programs in end-of-life care. The Johns Hopkins Nursing Leadership Academy for End of Life Care has also been established to improve nurses' knowledge of palliative care across nursing specialties. Under this initiative, nursing organizations have expressed a commitment to provide quality palliative care, and each has developed detailed plans regarding palliative care initiatives in their respective specialty.

National, state, and local indicators point to the need to prepare Advanced Practice Hospice and Palliative Nurses (APNs) who have advanced knowledge and skill in hospice and palliative care, who are competent to provide patient care across the life span, and who assume leadership roles in a variety of settings. APNs can play a vital role in palliative care by assessing, implementing, coordinating, and evaluating care throughout the disease trajectory, as well as by counseling and educating patients and families and facilitating continuity of care between hospital and home. Because of their proximity to patients, APNs are in ideal positions to assess, diagnose, and treat pain and other symptoms. APNs also identify ethical issues facing individuals and families, develop strategies to assist them in defining expected goals of care, and also access and coordinate appropriate care.

It is evident that palliative care is a rapidly developing specialty in medicine and nursing. Hospice and palliative care services, including inpatient palliative/hospice units, consultations teams, community or home hospice programs, ambulatory palliative care programs, and programs in skilled nursing facilities, are being developed across the country.

Professional Association and Certification

In 1987, the Hospice Nurses Association (HNA) was formed. This group became the first professional organization dedicated to promoting excellence in the practice of hospice nursing. Consistent with that goal, the HNA Board of Directors appointed the National Board for the Certification of Hospice Nurses (NBCHN) in 1992. In March of 1994, the NBCHN offered the first certification examination and the credential of Certified Registered Nurse Hospice (CRNH).

In 1997, recognizing the similarity in the nursing practice of the hospice nurse and the palliative nurse, the HNA expanded to embrace palliative nursing practice and became the Hospice and Palliative Nurses Association (HPNA). Hospice and palliative nurses were providing patient and family care in more diverse settings, and the fundamental nursing concepts developed in hospices were applied to other practice environments. The results of the 1998 Role Delineation Study, commissioned by the NBCHN, scientifically demonstrated that only minor differences in practice activity existed between end-of-life care offered by hospice nurses and palliative nurses working in nonhospice settings. These differences correlated with requirements of the role or practice setting.

In 1999 the NBCHN became the National Board for the Certification of Hospice and Palliative Nurses (NBCHPN®), offering a new professional certification designation to recognize base competence in hospice and palliative nursing—Certified Hospice and Palliative Nurse (CHPN). By early 2001, the number of credentialed nurses had risen to over 7,000. As end-of-life needs increase, the NBCHN seeks to provide the assurance of competency within those nursing agents who administer nursing care by revising the Statement of the Scope and Standard of Hospice and Palliative Nursing to address both the generalist and advanced practice nurse.

Scope of Hospice and Palliative Care Nursing Practice

The scope of hospice and palliative nursing continues to evolve as the science and art of palliative care develops. Hospice and palliative care nursing reflects a holistic philosophy of care implemented across the life span and across diverse health settings. Within a matrix of affiliation, including the patient and family, and other members of the interdisciplinary care team, hospice and palliative nurses provide evidence-based physical, emotional, psychosocial, and spiritual/existential care to individuals and families experiencing life-limiting progressive illness. The goal of hospice and palliative nursing is to promote the patient's quality of life through the relief of suffering along the illness trajectory, through the death of the patient, and into the bereavement period of the family. This goal is enhanced by completing the following activities:

- Comprehensive history: chief complaint, history of present illness, past medical/surgical history, family history, social history, immunization history, and allergies

- Review of systems

- Comprehensive physical and mental status examinations

- Determination of functional status

- Appropriate laboratory data and diagnostic studies or procedures

- Determination of effective and ineffective pharmacologic and nonpharmacologic therapies for symptom management

- Identification of past and present goals of care as stated by patient, surrogate, or healthcare proxy or as documented through advanced care planning

- Identification of health beliefs, values, and practices as related to culture, ethnicity, and religion/spirituality

- Recognition of response to advanced illness

- Determination of emotional status such as normal verses complicated grief, depression, anxiety, agitation, and terminal restlessness

- Identification of individual/family communication and coping patterns—past and present

- Assessment of patient and family support systems and environmental risks

- Determination of patient/family financial resources

- Spiritual assessment, including meaning of life, illness, and death, as well as a sense of hope/hopelessness, a need for forgiveness, fears, and a connectedness to self, others, nature, and God

Clinical Practice Setting

Hospice and palliative nursing is provided for patients and their families in a variety of care locations including, but not limited to, acute care hospital units; long-term care facilities; assisted living facilities; inpatient, home, or residential hospices; palliative care clinics or ambulatory settings; private practices; and prisons. Practice settings for hospice and palliative nursing are changing in response to the dynamic nature of today's healthcare environment.

Levels of Hospice and Palliative Nursing Practice

Hospice and palliative nurses are licensed registered nurses who are educationally prepared in nursing. Hospice and palliative nurses are qualified for specialty practice at two levels: generalist and advanced. These levels are differentiated by educational preparation, complexity of practice, and performance of certain nursing functions.

Generalist Level of Hospice and Palliative Nursing Practice

Registered nurses at the generalist level have completed a nursing program and passed the state licensure examination for registered nurses. Registered nurses who practice in hospice and palliative care settings may provide direct patient/family care and/or may function as educators, case managers, administrators, and in other nursing roles. Their practice should reflect the scope and standards of hospice and palliative nursing delineated in this document.

The generalist competencies in hospice and palliative care represent the knowledge, skills, and abilities demonstrated when providing evidence-based physical, emotional, psychosocial, and spiritual care (HPNA 2000). The care is provided in a collaborative manner across the life span in diverse settings to individuals and families experiencing life-limiting, progressive illness. The generalist level competencies and the related general statements are as follows:

Clinical Judgment

Clinical judgment at the hospice and palliative nurse generalist level is demonstrated in critical thinking, analysis, and clinical judgment in all aspects of hospice and palliative care of patients and families experiencing life-limiting illness. This includes use of the nursing process to address the physical, psychosocial, and spiritual needs of patients and families. The generalist and also the advanced practice hospice and palliative nurse must respond to all disease processes at the end of life including, but not limited to, neurological, cardiac, pulmonary, oncology, renal, dementias, diabetes, and HIV/AIDS. Clinical judgment is demonstrated in providing effective pain and symptom management.

Advocacy and Ethics

Advocacy and ethics at the hospice and palliative nurse generalist level incorporates ethical principles and professional standards in the care of patients and families experiencing life-limiting progressive illnesses and identifies and advocates for the patients' and families' wishes and preferences. Promoting ethical and legal decision making, advocating for personal wishes and preferences, ensuring access to care and community resources through influencing/developing health and social policy are ways to incorporate ethical principles and professional standards in the care of patients and families experiencing life-limiting, progressive illnesses.

Professionalism

Professionalism at the hospice and palliative nurse generalist level demonstrates knowledge, attitude, behavior, and skills that are consistent with the professional standards, code of ethics, and scope of practice for hospice and palliative nursing. Contributing to improved quality and cost-effective hospice and palliative services; participating in the generation, testing, and/or evaluation of hospice and palliative care knowledge and practice; and participating in the hospice and palliative care organizations are a few examples of professionalism demonstrated by the hospice and palliative care nurse.

Collaboration

Collaboration at the hospice and palliative nurse generalist level actively promotes dialogue with patients and families and facilitates collaborative practice with the healthcare team and community to address and plan for issues related to living with and dying from chronic, life-limiting, progressive illnesses through the bereavement phase.

Systems Thinking

Systems thinking at the hospice and palliative nurse generalist level utilizes system resources necessary to enhance the quality of life for patients and families experiencing life-limiting progressive illnesses through knowledge and negotiation.

Cultural Competence

Cultural competence at the hospice and palliative nurse generalist level demonstrates cultural competence by respecting and honoring the unique diversity and characteristics of patients, families, and colleagues in hospice and palliative care and bereavement. Cultural competence also includes hospice and palliative nurse behaviors that address psychosocial and spiritual needs of patient and family throughout the dying process and bereavement and incorporate cultural values and attitudes in developing the patient plan of care.

Facilitation of Learning

The hospice and palliative nurse promotes the learning of patient, family, self, members of the healthcare team, and community through the development, the implementation, and the evaluation of formal and informal education related to living with and dying from life-limiting progressive illnesses. This also includes creation of a healing environment to promote a peaceful death and the creation of opportunities and initiatives for the implementation of hospice and palliative care education for patients, families, colleagues, and community.

Communication

Communication at the hospice and palliative nurse generalist level demonstrates the use of effective verbal, nonverbal, and written communication with patients and families, members of the healthcare team, and community in order to therapeutically address and accurately convey the hospice and palliative care needs of patients and families throughout the disease process and bereavement. Communication at the generalist level includes the utilization of therapeutic communication skills in all interactions to support those who are experiencing loss, grief, and bereavement.

Advanced Practice Level of Hospice and Palliative Nursing Practice

Advanced practice hospice and palliative nursing is an emerging role in response to individual, professional, and societal needs related to the experience of life-limiting progressive illness. The Advanced Practice Hospice and Palliative Nurse is a registered nurse (RN) who is educationally prepared at the master's level or higher in nursing as a Clinical Nurse Specialist (CNS) or Nurse Practitioner (NP). An Advanced Practice Hospice and Palliative Nurse:

- Has the knowledge, skills and aptitudes to perform all aspects of basic hospice and palliative nursing as well as the skills to perform the advanced-level care responsibilities.

- Is distinguished by the ability to synthesize complex data, implement advanced plans of care, and provide leadership in hospice and palliative care.

The roles of the Advanced Practice Hospice and Palliative Nurse include, but are not limited to, expert clinician, leader/facilitator of interdisciplinary teams, educator, researcher, consultant, collaborator, advocate, and/or administrator.

Advanced Practice Hospice and Palliative Nurses who have fulfilled the requirements established by their state nurse practice acts may be authorized to assume autonomous responsibility for clinical role functions, which may include prescription of controlled substances, medications, or therapies. To practice as an advanced practice hospice and palliative nurse, national certification in advanced practice hospice and palliative nursing is recommended, although it is recognized that the advanced practice hospice and palliative nurse may have concurrent advanced practice certification in another specialty.

Standards of Hospice and Palliative Nursing

The standards of hospice and palliative nursing practice are authoritative statements described by the Hospice and Palliative Nurses Association for the nursing profession, which identifies the responsibilities for which hospice and palliative nurses are accountable. The standards reflect the values and priorities of hospice and palliative nursing and provide a framework for the evaluation of practice. The standards are written in measurable terms and define the hospice and palliative nurses' accountability to the public and the patient/family outcomes for which they are responsible.

The standards are divided into two sections: the Standards of Care and the Standards of Professional Performance. Each section has identified criteria that allow the standards to be measured. The criteria include key indicators of competent practice. The standards remain stable over time as they reflect the philosophical values of the profession. However, the criteria should be revised to incorporate advancements in scientific knowledge, technology, and clinical practice. The criteria must be consistent with current nursing practice and reflect evidence-based practice.

Standards of Care

Standards of care describe a competent level of generalist and advanced practice registered nursing care, as demonstrated by the nursing process, involving assessment, diagnosis, outcomes identification, planning, implementation, and evaluation. The development of a therapeutic nurse–patient/family relationship is essential throughout the nursing process. The nursing process forms the foundation of clinical decision-making and encompasses all significant actions taken by hospice and palliative care nurses in providing care to individuals and families. Several themes of nursing practice provide additional dimensions for attention, such as:

- Providing age-appropriate, culturally, ethnically, and spiritually sensitive care and support
- Maintaining a safe environment
- Educating patients and families to identify appropriate settings and treatment options
- Assuring continuity of care
- Coordinating the care across all settings and among caregivers
- Managing information
- Communicating effectively

Standards of Professional Performance

Standards of professional performance and the associated measurement criteria describe competent professional role behaviors, including activities related to quality of care, performance appraisal, education, collegiality, ethics, collaboration, research, and resource utilization. Hospice and palliative should be self-directed and purposeful in seeking necessary knowledge and skills to develop and maintain their competency. The hospice and palliative nurses' professionalism may be enhanced through membership in their professional organizations, certification in their specialty, and professional development through academic and continuing education.

STANDARDS OF CARE

STANDARD 1. ASSESSMENT
The hospice and palliative nurse collects basic individual and family data.

Measurement Criteria

1. The priority of data collection is determined by the patient's and family's immediate condition or needs.

2. Data are collected in collaboration with the patient, family, healthcare providers, or from community agencies, as well as from past and current medical records.

3. Data collection may involve the use of various assessment techniques and standardized instruments, as appropriate.

4. The assessment process, employing critical thinking, analysis, and judgment, is systematic and ongoing.

5. The data are synthesized and prioritized.

6. Relevant data are documented in a retrievable form.

7. Assessment data are collected at either a generalist or advanced level based on the educational preparation and clinical expertise of hospice and palliative nurses, who utilize research and other evidence to guide their assessment knowledge.

Additional measurement criteria for the advanced practice hospice and palliative nurse:

(a) In-depth and comprehensive assessments are conducted based on a synthesis of individual and family health;

(b) A ssessments are based on advanced knowledge; and

(c) Diagnostic tests and procedures relevant to the individuals' current status are initiated and integrated.

STANDARD 2. DIAGNOSIS
The hospice and palliative nurse analyzes the assessment data in determining diagnoses utilizing an accepted framework that supports hospice and palliative nursing knowledge.

Measurement Criteria

Diagnoses are:

1. Derived from the analyses of the multidimensional assessment data.

2. Validated with the patient, family, and interdisciplinary team members and other healthcare providers when possible and appropriate.

3. Based on actual or potential responses to alterations in health.

4. Used to identify problems that may be resolved, diminished, or prevented through nursing and/or interdisciplinary intervention.

5. Documented in a manner that facilitates determination of expected outcomes and plan of care.

6. Communicated to other interdisciplinary team members or consultants.

Additional measurement criteria for the advanced practice hospice and palliative nurse:

(a) Based on critical analysis of the data, additional diagnostic tests and procedures are initiated to complete the diagnostic analysis;

(b) Diagnoses are derived and prioritized diagnoses from the assessment data based on appropriate, complex, clinical reasoning;

(c) A differential diagnosis is formulated by systematically comparing and contrasting clinical findings; and

(d) Diagnoses are made by conducting a critical analysis and synthesis of information obtained during the interview, physical examination, and diagnostic tests or diagnostic procedures.

STANDARD 3. OUTCOME IDENTIFICATION
The hospice and palliative nurse identifies expected outcomes relevant to the individual and family, in partnership with the interdisciplinary/healthcare team.

Measurement Criteria

1. Expected outcomes are derived from the diagnoses.

2. Expected outcomes are mutually formulated with the individual, family, other members of the interdisciplinary/healthcare team, and other health providers, when possible and appropriate.

3. Expected outcomes are culturally appropriate and reflective of the individuals' and families' values, beliefs, and preferences.

4. Expected outcomes are realistic in relation to the individuals' and families' goals of care and are developed to improve quality of life.

5. Expected outcomes are patient-oriented, evidence-based, realistic, and cost-effective.

6. Expected outcomes are attainable in relation to the prognosis of the individual and the resources available.

7. Expected outcomes provide direction of continuity of care across all care settings, from admission through family bereavement.

8. Expected outcomes include a time estimate for attainment and are documented as measurable goals.

Additional measurement criteria for the advanced practice hospice and palliative nurse:

Expected outcomes are:

(a) Based on a critical analysis of both complex assessment data and diagnoses that are relevant to the individual and family, and the interdisciplinary/healthcare team, when appropriate;

(b) Identified, with consideration of associated risks, benefits, and costs;

(c) Developed that are consistent with current scientific and clinical practice knowledge; and

(d) Modified based on changes in the individuals' and families' health status.

Appendix A: Hospice and Palliative Nursing Practice (2002)   **73**

STANDARD **4.** PLANNING
The hospice and palliative nurse develops a plan of care—a plan negotiated among the individual, family, and interdisciplinary/healthcare team—that includes interventions and treatments to attain expected outcomes.

Measurement Criteria

1. The plan of care is individualized to the persons' and families' physical, emotional, psychosocial, cultural, and spiritual needs, desires, and resources.

2. The plan of care is developed in collaboration with the individual and family, other members of the interdisciplinary/healthcare team, and other healthcare providers as appropriate.

3. The plan of care is evidence-based and consistent with current hospice and palliative care practice.

4. The plan provides for continuity of care across all care settings, from admission through family bereavement.

5. The plan of care is dynamic, documented, and updated regularly as the patient and family status and priorities change.

Additional measurement criteria for the advanced practice hospice and palliative nurse:

The comprehensive plan of care

(a) Prescribes evidence-based interventions to attain expected outcomes and reviews with individuals and families the relative risks, benefits, burdens, and costs of interventions;

(b) Describes and documents the assessment/diagnostic strategies and therapeutic interventions that reflect current healthcare knowledge, research, and practice;

(c) Reflects their responsibilities and the responsibilities of the individual, family, and other members of the interdisciplinary/healthcare team;

(d) Addresses strategies for promotion of quality of life through independent clinical decision making; and

(e) Provides direction to other members of the interdisciplinary/ healthcare team.

STANDARD 5. IMPLEMENTATION
The hospice and palliative nurse implements the interventions identified in the plan of care.

Measurement Criteria

1. Interventions are selected based on the available resources and the values, preferences, and goals of the individual, and family.

2. Interventions are implemented in a safe, timely, ethical, and culturally competent manner.

3. Interventions are implemented in a collaborative manner with other members of the interdisciplinary/healthcare team.

4. Interventions are evidence-based.

5. Interventions are modified based on continued assessment of the individuals' and families' response to care and other clinical indicators.

6. Interventions are documented in a format that is related to individual/family outcomes, accessible to the interdisciplinary/ healthcare team, and retrievable for future data analysis and research.

7. The wide range of interventions, which involve either the provision of direct care, consultation, referral, or case management to promote quality of life for individuals and families, may include, but are not limited to, the following interventions:

   (a) Facilitation of self-care to promote physical, emotional, social, and spiritual well-being;

   (b) Maximizing, restoring, and maintaining functional status to promote activities of daily living, as appropriate to the individual and the enhancement of well-being;

   (c) Health promotion and maintenance to prevent or limit disease progression and the development of other physical or emotional illnesses;

continued

(d) Health teaching to achieve satisfying, productive, and healthy patterns of living that recognizes the individuals' and families' developmental level, culture, learning needs, readiness and ability to learn, and barriers;

(e) Counseling and psychological interventions to improve or regain previous coping abilities, foster emotional and spiritual health, and prevent mental illness and disability;

(f) Pharmacologic, nonpharmacologic, and complementary therapies to provide symptom management and the relief of suffering; and

(g) Advocacy to promote self-determination, resolve conflicts, and ensure ethically appropriate care.

Additional measurement criteria for the advanced practice hospice and palliative nurse includes prescribing, ordering, or implementing interventions related to the following:

(a) *Case Management and Coordination of Care*

- Uses sophisticated data synthesis with consideration of the individuals' and families' complex needs and desired outcomes, and

- Negotiates health-related services and additional specialized care with the individual and family and appropriate systems, agencies, and provider.

(b) *Consultation*

- Influences the plan of care for individuals and families experiencing life-limiting, progressive illness; and

- Enhances the abilities of others and effects change in the system based on the application of theory, recognition of mutual respect, delineation of role responsibilities, and facilitation of the communication of recommendations.

(c) *Health Promotion, Health Maintenance, and Health Teaching*

- Employs complex strategies, interventions, and teaching methodologies based on assessment of risks, epidemiologic principles, learning theory, and the individuals' and families' health beliefs and practices.

(d) *Prescriptive Authority and Treatment*

- Uses prescriptive authority, procedures, and treatments in accordance with state and federal laws and regulations to treat symptoms, maintain or improve functional status, or provide preventative care.

(e) *Referral*

- Identifies the need for additional care and makes appropriate referrals;

- Facilitates continuity of care by implementing recommendations from referral sources; and

- Refers directly to specific providers based on individual and family needs with consideration of benefits, burdens, costs, and goals of care.

STANDARD 6. EVALUATION
The hospice and palliative nurse evaluates the individuals' and families' progress in attaining expected outcomes.

Measurement Criteria

1. Evaluation is systematic, criterion-based, ongoing, and reviewed with other members of the interdisciplinary/healthcare team.

2. The effectiveness of interventions in relation to the expected outcomes is evaluated, using standardized methods, as appropriate.

3. The evaluation process, to ascertain the level of satisfaction, includes collaboration of the individual, family, and other members of the interdisciplinary/healthcare team collaborate in the evaluation process to ascertain the level of satisfaction with care, and their evaluatation the benefits, burdens, and costs associated with the plan of care.

4. Ongoing assessment data are used to revise diagnoses, expected outcomes, and the plan of care as needed.

5. Revisions in the diagnoses, expected outcomes, and the plan of care are documented and communicated to the individual, family, and other members of the interdisciplinary/healthcare team to ensure continuity of care.

Additional measurement criteria for the advanced practice hospice and palliative nurse:

The evaluation process :

(a) Includes critical appraisal of all relevant and available data related to the attainment of expected outcomes;

(b) Incorporates advanced knowledge, practice, and research into the evaluation process; and

(c) Includes responsibility for the overall evaluation, revision, documentation, and communication of the plan within the healthcare settings.

Standards of Professional Performance

Standard 1. Quality of Care
The hospice and palliative nurse systematically evaluates the quality and effectiveness of hospice and palliative nursing practice.

Measurement Criteria

1. The hospice and palliative nurse participates in quality care activities as appropriate to the individual's position, education, and practice environment. Such activities may include:

   (a) Participation on teams that evaluate interdisciplinary clinical practice caring for patients and families;

   (b) Identification of aspects of care important for quality monitoring;

   (c) Identification of indicators used to monitor quality and effectiveness of nursing care;

   (d) Seeking feedback from the patient and significant others about quality and outcomes of the patient's care;

   (e) Analysis of quality data to identify opportunities for improving care;

   (f) Formulation of recommendations to improve palliative care nursing;

   (g) Development of policies, procedures, and practice guidelines to improve quality of care; and

   (h) Implementation of activities to enhance the quality of nursing practice.

2. The hospice and palliative nurse participates in quality-of-life care activities in a coordinated and collaborative manner.

3. The hospice and palliative nurse uses the results of quality-of-care activities to initiate changes in practice or redesign processes.

4. The hospice and palliative nurse uses the results of quality-of-life care activities to initiate changes impacting end-of life care throughout the healthcare delivery system.

Additional measurement criteria for the advanced practice hospice and palliative nurse:

(a) Develops criteria for and evaluates the quality of care and effectiveness of advanced hospice and palliative practice nursing.

(b) Assumes a leadership role in establishing and monitoring standards of practice to improve patient and family care;

(c) Utilizes the results of quality-of-care activities to initiative changes throughout the healthcare system, as appropriate;

(d) Participates in efforts to minimize costs and unnecessary duplication of testing or other diagnostic activities and to facilitate timely treatment of the patient and family;

(e) Analyzes factors related to safety, satisfaction, effectiveness, and cost/benefit options with the client and other providers as appropriate;

(f) Analyzes organizational systems for barriers and promoting enhancements that affect patient and family healthcare status;

(g) Bases evaluations on current knowledge, practice, and research; and

(h) Seeks professional certification in advanced hospice and palliative care when available.

STANDARD 2. PERFORMANCE APPRAISAL
The hospice and palliative nurse evaluates one's own nursing practice in relation to professional practice standards and relevant statutes and regulations.

Measurement Criteria

1. The hospice and palliative nurse engages in a personal performance appraisal on a regular basis, identifying areas of strengths as well as areas for professional/practice development.

2. The hospice and palliative nurse seeks constructive feedback regarding one's own practice and role performance from peers, professional colleagues, patients, families, and others.

3. The hospice and palliative nurse takes action to achieve goals identified during performance appraisals and peer review, resulting in changes in practice and role performance.

4. The hospice and palliative nurse participates in peer review as appropriate.

5. The hospice and palliative nurse's practice reflects knowledge of current practice standards, laws, and regulations.

Additional measurement criteria for the advanced practice hospice and palliative nurse:

(a) Evaluates one's own practice and the practice of subordinates in regard to institutional, state, and federal laws and regulations as well as patient, family, community, and environmental outcomes related to the potential or actual process and treatments;

(b) Seeks routine feedback regarding one's own practice and role performance from peers, professional colleagues, members of the healthcare team, and patients receiving care;

(c) Identifies areas of strength and areas for further development, modifies practice in response to this evaluation, and obtains necessary education and/or assistance to meet learning/performance goals; and

(d) Participates in appraisal of peer performance to further strengthen overall healthcare team performance and effectiveness, communicating areas of concern to peers and/or appropriate management personnel for further action.

STANDARD 3. EDUCATION
The hospice and palliative nurse acquires and maintains current knowledge and competency in hospice and palliative care nursing.

Measurement Criteria

1. The hospice and palliative nurse participates in ongoing educational activities related to clinical knowledge and professional issues.

2. The hospice and palliative nurse seeks experiences to develop, maintain, or refine clinical competence.

continued

3. The hospice and palliative nurse acquires additional knowledge and skills appropriate to palliative care nursing by participating in educational programs and activities, conferences, workshops, and interdisciplinary professional meetings.

4. The hospice and palliative nurse documents one's own educational activities.

Additional measurement criteria for the advanced practice hospice and palliative nurse:

(a) Acquires and maintains knowledge related to current research, scientific findings, and advanced clinical practice in the area of hospice and palliative care nursing and related disciplines;

(b) Utilizes current research and scientific findings and participates in ongoing educational activities to expand advanced clinical knowledge and to enhance role performance;

(c) Maintains expected education, certification, and licensure requirements in accordance with institutional, state, and federal laws and regulations as well as the requirements of specialty nursing certification organizations;

(d) Updates one's own knowledge of political, cultural, spiritual, social, professional, and ethical issues as related to advanced practice palliative care nursing and shares knowledge with others; and

(e) Seeks additional experiences to maintain and expand areas of advanced practice hospice and palliative nursing expertise.

STANDARD 4. COLLEGIALITY
The hospice and palliative nurse interacts with and contributes to the professional development of peers and other healthcare providers as colleagues.

Measurement Criteria

1. The hospice and palliative nurse uses opportunities in practice to exchange knowledge, skills, and clinical observations with colleagues and others.

2. The hospice and palliative nurse provides peers with constructive feedback regarding their practice.

3. The hospice and palliative nurse assists others in identifying teaching/learning needs related to clinical care, role performance, and professional development.

4. The hospice and palliative nurse contributes to an environment that is conducive to the clinical education of nursing students, other healthcare students, and other members of the interdisciplinary team as appropriate.

5. The hospice and palliative nurse contributes to a supportive and healthy work environment.

6. The hospice and palliative nurse serves as a consultant on palliative care issues to other healthcare providers, agencies, and the community at large.

7. The hospice and palliative nurse participates in the development of educational programs for nursing peers, interdisciplinary team members, and the community at large.

8. The hospice and palliative nurse accurately differentiates the scope and function of each member of the interdisciplinary/healthcare team.

Additional measurement criteria for the advanced practice hospice and palliative nurse:

(a) Serves as a leader, mentor, and role model for the professional development of peers, colleagues, and others;

(b) Contributes to the professional development and education of others to improve patient, family, community, and environmental outcomes as well as to improve his or her professional growth, especially in the areas of advanced practice hospice and palliative care nursing;

(c) Actively participates in professional and specialty nursing organizations such as the Hospice and Palliative Nurses Association;

(d) Publishes and shares knowledge through presentations at professional meetings to contribute to hospice and palliative care nursing;

continued

(e) Serves as a role model, preceptor, mentor, and facilitator of learning in generalist hospice and palliative care nursing and advanced practice hospice and palliative care nursing;

(f) Contributes to the identification of future educational and research ideas as well as to the development of creative and innovative ways to improve care delivery and outcomes in hospice and palliative care; and

(g) Serves as a liaison to institutional, local, state, and national legislative bodies to be influential regarding issues relating to advanced practice hospice and palliative care nursing with the goal of improved outcomes for the patient, family, community, and environment related to the potential or actual disease process and treatments.

STANDARD 5. ETHICS
The hospice and palliative nurse demonstrates moral discernment, critical reasoning, and discriminating judgment in integrating ethics into hospice and palliative nursing during all interactions with the patient, family, organization, and community.

Measurement Criteria

1. The hospice and palliative nurse acts in accordance with the current *Code of Ethics for Nurses with Interpretive Statements* (ANA, 2001) and other position statements that guide the palliative care nurse's practice.

2. The hospice and palliative nurse maintains patient and family confidentiality within legal, ethical, and regulatory parameters.

3. The hospice and palliative nurse acts as a patient and family advocate and assists the patient and family in developing skills so that they can advocate for themselves.

4. The hospice and palliative nurse delivers care in a nonjudgmental and nondiscriminatory manner that is sensitive to patient and family diversity.

5. The hospice and palliative nurse delivers care in a manner that preserves/protects patient and family autonomy, dignity, and rights.

6. The hospice and palliative nurse collaborates with the members of the interdisciplinary/healthcare team and seeks other available resources to help in the formulation of ethical decisions.

7. The hospice and palliative nurse recognizes one's own values and beliefs when assisting in the formulation of ethical decisions.

8. The hospice and palliative nurse seeks to prevent ethical problems, identifies ethical dilemmas that occur within the practice environment, and seeks available resources to help resolve ethical dilemmas.

9. The hospice and palliative nurse reports abuse of patients' rights and incompetent, unethical, and illegal practices.

10. The hospice and palliative nurse participates in the informed consent process (including the right to refuse) for patients' procedures, tests, treatments, and research participation, as appropriate.

11. The hospice and palliative nurse maintains and updates one's own knowledge of ethical issues.

12. The hospice and palliative nurse recognizes and accepts an interactive relationship with the patient and family, which includes the recognition and maintenance of professional boundaries.

Additional measurement criteria for the advanced practice hospice and palliative nurse:

(a) Emphasizes to nursing colleagues the importance of the *Code of Ethics for Nurses with Interpretative Statements* (ANA, 2001), and other professional position statements;

(b) Instructs, mentors, and models for others through integrating ethical conduct into one's own her or his professional practice;

(c) Facilitates the development of professional and moral conscience in colleagues;

(d) Ensures that the rights of the patient, family, community, and nurses are respected and safeguarded;

(e) Provides education and information to the patient and family to facilitate informed decision making, including information about advanced directives and participation in clinical trials;

continued

(f) Ensures that the patient, family, nurses, other professional colleagues, and the community discuss and participate in resolving ethical dilemmas;

(g) Recognizes ethical dilemmas that confront the patient, family, nurses, and other professional colleagues and actively supports those involved in resolving the dilemmas;

(h) Facilitates case analyses by articulating to the interdisciplinary/healthcare team a process for moral reasoning;

(i) Uses and assists the patient, family, community, and professional colleagues in accessing the formal mechanism for resolving ethical dilemmas;

(j) Assists in ensuring that the institution's policies and procedures, protocols, guidelines, and/or standards uphold and enhance ethical practice;

(k) Participates in educational programs that identify and support discussion of moral and ethical issues; and

(l) Strives to maintain the integrity of the profession and to enhance the professionalism and culture of nursing in all settings.

STANDARD 6. COLLABORATION
The hospice and palliative nurse collaborates with patient and family, members of the interdisciplinary/healthcare team, and other healthcare providers in providing patient and family care.

Measurement Criteria

1. The hospice and palliative nurse communicates with the patient and family, other members of the interdisciplinary/healthcare team, and other healthcare providers regarding patient and family care and the nursing role in the provision of hospice and palliative care.

2. The hospice and palliative nurse collaborates with the patient and family, members of the interdisciplinary/healthcare team, and other healthcare providers in the formulation of overall goals, plan of care, and decisions related to the delivery of services.

3. The hospice and palliative nurse consults with and is a consultant to members of the interdisciplinary/healthcare team and other healthcare providers for patient and family care, as needed.

4. The hospice and palliative nurse coordinates the implementation of care provided for the patient and family by the interdisciplinary/healthcare team.

5. The hospice and palliative nurse makes referrals, including provisions for continuity of care when appropriate.

6. The hospice and palliative nurse collaborates with other disciplines in teaching, consultation, management, and research activities.

Additional measurement criteria for the advanced practice hospice and palliative nurse:

(a) Promotes an interdisciplinary/healthcare team approach to providing advanced practice hospice and palliative nursing to the patient, family, community, and environment related to the potential or actual disease process and treatments;

(b) Consults with other disciplines and members of the interdisciplinary/healthcare team to maximize advanced palliative care nursing as related to health education, health promotion, health restoration, and/or health maintenance;

(c) Collaborates with other disciplines and members of the interdisciplinary/healthcare team regarding continuity of care, rehabilitation, home care, and symptom management; and

(d) Participates in establishing clinical practice guidelines, including clinical pathways, algorithms for symptom management, and practice protocols.

STANDARD 7. RESEARCH
The hospice and palliative nurse uses research findings in practice.

Measurement Criteria

1. The hospice and palliative nurse utilizes research and other evidences to develop the plan of care and interventions.

continued

2. The hospice and palliative nurse participates in research activities as appropriate to the individual's position, education, and practice environment. Such activities may include:

(a) Consulting with research colleagues and experts;

(b) Identifying clinical problems suitable for hospice and palliative care research or interdisciplinary research;

(c) Participating in development of a research plan;

(d) Participating in data collection and analysis;

(e) Communicating and disseminating findings;

(f) Critiquing and evaluating research findings for application to practice;

(g) Utilizing research findings to assist in the development of policies, protocols, procedures, and guidelines for hospice and palliative care; and

(h) Sharing research findings with others through discussion groups, professional presentations, and publications.

Additional measurement criteria for the advanced practice hospice and palliative nurse:

(a) Utilizes research to identify, examine, validate, and evaluate knowledge, theories, and creative approaches to health care related to advanced practice hospice and palliative nursing practice with the goal of improved outcomes for the patient, family, community, and environment;

(b) Examines, validates, and evaluates current hospice and palliative nursing practice in regard to current research findings and develops potential research topics and testable hypotheses;

(c) Promotes hospice and palliative nurses' interest in basic and clinical research relevant to hospice and palliative care and involves staff in identification, data collection, and modification of practice based on research findings;

(d) Collaborates with colleagues and other members of the interdisciplinary/healthcare team in the identification, development, implementation, and utilization of research findings;

(e) Disseminates relevant research findings through practice, education, and consultation;

(f) Ensures that institutional safeguards are intact to protect the rights of human subjects and upholds these rights in daily practice; and

(g) Conducts or participates in writing proposals, conducting research, and disseminating findings through oral and written presentations. If doctorally prepared, pursues funding sources and conducts and disseminates research to improve hospice and palliative patient care and/or advance the science of nursing.

STANDARD 8. RESOURCE UTILIZATION
The hospice and palliative nurse considers factors related to safety, effectiveness, and cost in planning and delivering patient and family care.

Measurement Criteria

1. The hospice and palliative nurse evaluates factors related to safety, effectiveness, and cost when two or more practice options would result in the same expected patient and family outcomes.

2. The hospice and palliative nurse assists the patient and family with identifying and securing appropriate services available to address health-related needs.

3. The hospice and palliative nurse assigns or delegates tasks, as defined by the state nurse practice acts, and according to the knowledge and skills of the designated caregiver.

4. The hospice and palliative nurse assigns or delegates tasks based on the needs and conditions of the patient and family, the potential for harm, the stability of the patient's condition, the complexity of the task, and the predictability of the outcome.

5. The hospice and palliative nurse assists the patient and family in becoming informed consumers about the costs, risks, and benefits of treatment and end-of-life care.

6. The hospice and palliative nurse documents the effects of resource utilization and changing patterns of healthcare delivery on hospice and palliative care nursing and patient/family outcomes.

Additional measurement criteria for the advanced practice hospice and palliative nurse:

(a) Seeks to provide cost-effective, quality care by using the most appropriate resources and delegating care to the most appropriate, qualified healthcare clinician;

(b) Identifies the most appropriate settings for the delivery of hospice and palliative care consistent with the goals, preferences, and needs of patients and families experiencing life-limiting, progressive illness; and

(c) Assists patients and families in accessing and utilizing resources needed for quality care across hospice and palliative care settings.

GLOSSARY

Admission process. An activity that begins with the initial referral to the program of care and continues through to the development of the interdisciplinary plan of care.

Assessment. A systematic, dynamic process in which the nurse, through interaction with the patient and family, significant others, and other members of the interdisciplinary/healthcare team or consultants collect and analyze data about the patient and family. Data may include physical, psychological, sociocultural, spiritual, cognitive, functional, developmental, economic, and lifestyle dimensions.

Continuity of care. An interdisciplinary process that includes patients and significant others in the development of a coordinated plan of care. This process facilitates the patient's transition between settings, based on changing needs and available resources.

Criteria. Relevant, measurable indicators of the standards of hospice and palliative care nursing practice.

Diagnosis. A clinical judgment about the patient's and family's response to actual or potential health conditions or needs. Diagnoses provide the basis for determination of a plan of care to achieve expected outcomes.

Evaluation. The process of determining both the patient's and family's progress toward the attainment of expected outcomes and the effectiveness of nursing care with consideration for the patient's value system and goals for care.

Family. Includes not only persons bound by biological or legal ties, but also those who define themselves as a "close other" with another person, or "those who function in familistic ways" (Settles, 1987, p. 160). These ways of functioning can include nurturance, intimacy, companionship, and economic, social, psychosocial, and physical support in time of need or in illness (Matocha, 1992).

Healthcare providers. Individuals with special expertise who provide healthcare services or assistance to patients. They must include nurses, physicians, psychologists, social workers, nutritionists/dietitians, and various therapists and other members of the interdisciplinary team.

Implementation. May include any or all of the following activities: teaching, intervening, delegating, and coordinating. The patient and family or other members of the interdisciplinary/healthcare team may be designated to implement interventions within the plan of care.

Interdisciplinary team. A highly qualified, specially trained team of hospice and palliative care professionals and volunteers who work together to meet the physiological, psychological, social, spiritual, and economic needs of the patient and family facing terminal illness and bereavement. The team may include physicians, nurses, social workers, clergy, bereavement counselors, and other members as indicated for specific needs.

Nurse. An individual who is licensed by a state agency to practice as a registered nurse.

Nursing. The diagnosis and treatment of human responses to actual or potential health problems.

Outcomes. Measurable expected patient and family-focused goals that translate into observable behaviors.

Palliative Care Continuum. Palliative care provides support and care for persons and their families experiencing life-limiting, progressive illness from the time of diagnosis with advanced disease, through the death of the person, and into the bereavement period of the family. The goal is to promote the best possible quality of life for patients and families so that they may live as fully and comfortably as possible. Palliative care recognizes dying as part of the normal process of living and focuses on maintaining the quality of remaining life. Palliative care affirms life and neither hastens nor postpones death. Palliative care exist in the hope and belief that through appropriate care, and the promotion of a caring community sensitive to their needs, patients and their families may be free to attain a degree of mental and spiritual preparation for death that is satisfactory to them. Hospice care is the final portion of the Palliative Care Continuum regulated by Medicare as a 6-month period if the disease runs its normal course.

Patient. Recipient of nursing care. The term patient is used in the Standards to provide consistency and brevity, bearing in mind that the terms client or individual might be better choices in some instances. When the patient is an individual client, the focus is on the health state, problems, or needs of the single person. When the patient is a family or group, the focus is on the health state of the unit as a whole or the reciprocal effects of an individual's health state on the other members of the unit.

Plan of care. Comprehensive outline of care, written according to the patient/family wishes and intended to attain expected outcomes when implemented by the interdisciplinary team.

Resources. Assets that can be drawn upon by the patient and family for aid. Types of resources include, but are not limited to, financial, emotional, spiritual, social, psychological, and physical.

Standard. Authoritative statement enunciated and promulgated by the profession by which the quality of practice, service, or education can be judged.

Standards of care. Authoritative statements that describe a competent level of clinical nursing practice demonstrated through assessment, diagnosis, outcome identification, planning, implementation, and planning.

Standards of nursing practice. Authoritative statements that describe a level of care or performance common to the profession of nursing by which the quality of nursing practice can be judged. Standards of clinical nursing practice include both standards of care and standards of professional performance.

Standards of professional performance. Authoritative statements that describe a competent level of behavior in the professional role, including activities related to quality of care performance appraisal, education, collegiality, ethics, collaboration, research, and resource utilization.

Unit of care. The terminally ill patient and their family. The patient and family are an interdependent, integrated whole composed of two or more individuals. They experience individual as well as over lapping needs.

REFERENCES

AACN (American Association of Colleges of Nursing). (1997). *Peaceful death document.* Washington D.C.: Roundtable Discussion on Palliative Care. Washington, D.C.

ANA (American Association of Nurses). (2001). *Code of ethics for nurses with interpretive statements.* Washington, D.C.: American Nurses Publishing.

Billings, J. A., & Block, S. (1997). Palliative care in undergraduate medical education. *Journal of the American Medical Association* 278 (9), 733–736.

Dahlin, C. (1999). Access to Hospice. In I. Corless & Z. Foster (Eds.). *The Hospice Heritage: Celebrating the future* (pp. 75–84). New York: The Haworth Press, Inc.

Doyle, D., Hanks, G., & MacDonald, N. (1998). *Oxford textbook of palliative medicine.* New York: Oxford Medical Publication.

Ferris, F., & Cummings, I. (1995). *Palliative care: Towards a consensus in standardized principles of practice.* Ottawa, Ontario: Canadian Palliative Care Association.

Field, M., & Cassel, C. (1997). *Approaching death: improving care at the end of life.* Washington, DC: National Academy Press.

Knaus, W. et al. (1995). A controlled trial to improve care for seriously ill hospitalized patients. *Journal of the America Medical Association* 274 (20), 1591–1598. HPNA (Hospice and Palliative Nurses Association). (2002). *Competencies For advance practice hospice and palliative care nurses.* Kendall-Hunt.

———. (2002). *Professional competencies for generalist hospice and palliative nurses.* Kendall-Hunt.

Matocha, L. K. (1992). Case study interviews: Caring for person with AIDS. In J. F. Gilgun, K. Daly, & G. Handel (Eds.), *Quantitative methods in family research* (pp. 66–84). Newbury Park, California.

Last Acts Task Force. (1998). National policy statements on end of life care: Precepts of palliative care. *Journal of Palliative Medicine 1*, 109–112.

Portenoy, R., & Bruera, B. (1997). *Topics in palliative care: Volume 1.* New York: Oxford Medical Publications.

Randall, F., & Downie, R. S. (1996). *Palliative care ethics.* New York: Oxford Medical Publications.

Settles, B. H. (1987). A perspective on tomorrow's families. In M. B. Sussman & S. K. S. K. Steinmetz (Eds.), *Handbook of marriage and the family* (pp. 157–180). New York: Plenum.

Sherman, D. W. (2001). Access to hospice care. *Journal of Palliative Medicine, 3*(4), 407–411.

Index

Pages in the 2002 *Scope and Standards of Hospice and Palliative Nursing Practice* are marked by brackets [ ].

Body of knowledge (*continued*)
  evaluation and, [78]
  implementation and, 18
  outcomes identification and, 14, 15, [73]
  planning and, 17, [74]
  prescriptive authority and treatment, 23
  professional practice evaluation and, [81]
  quality of practice and, 27, 28, [80]
  research and, 39, 40, [88]

C
Care recipient. *See* Patient
Care standards. *See* Standards of practice
Case management. *See* Coordination of care
Certification and credentialing, *xi, xii, xiii,* 9, [70]
  advanced practice, 6, [68]
  education and, [82]
  generalist practice, 3, [65]
  leadership and, 43
  quality of practice and, 28, [80]
Certified Hospice and Palliative Nurse (CHPN), *xiii,* [63]
Certified Registered Nurse Hospice (CRNH), *xii, xiii,* [63]
Client. *See* Patient
Clinical judgment, 3, [66]
  See also Critical thinking, analysis, and synthesis
Clinical Nurse Specialist (CNS), *ix,* 5, [60, 68]
Clinical settings. *See* Practice settings
Code of Ethics for Nurses with Interpretive Statements, 37, [84, 85]
  See also Ethics
Collaboration, 4, 9, [70]
  advanced practice, 6, [68]
  generalist practice, 3, [66, 67]
  ethics and, [85]
  evaluation and, [77]
  implementation and, 18, [75]
  planning and, 17, [74]
  quality of practice and, [79]
  research and, [88]

standard of professional performance, 35–36, [86–87]
  See also Healthcare providers; Interdisciplinary health care
Collegiality, 9, [70]
  consultation and, 22
  cultural competence and, [67]
  diagnosis and, 13
  education and, 5, 29, [67]
  ethics and, 37, [85, 86]
  implementation and, 18
  professional practice evaluation and, 31, 32, [80, 81]
  research and, [88]
  standard of professional performance, 33–34, [82–84]
Communication, *x,* 2, 4, 5, 8, [67–68, 70]
  assessment and, 11, [65]
  collaboration and, 35, 36
  collegiality and, 33, [83]
  consultation and, 22, [76]
  diagnosis and, 13, [72]
  education and, 29, [82]
  evaluation and, 24, [77, 78]
  leadership and, 44
  outcomes identification and, 14
  planning and, 16
  research and, 39, 40, [88, 89]
Community resources
  collaboration and, 4, [67]
  coordination of care and, 20
  implementation and, 18
  resource utilization and, 41
Competence assessment. *See* Certification and credentialing
Competencies, *xi*
  advanced practice level, *ix,* 5–6, [68]
  general practice level, 3–5, [65–68]
Confidentiality, 8, 37
  See also Ethics
Consultation, 6
  collaboration and, 36
  implementation and, 7
  planning and, 17
  standard of practice, 22, [76]
Continuity of care, *xii,* 8, [62, 70]
  collaboration and, 35, [87]

communication and, 5, [67]
consultation and, 22
coordination of care and, 20, [76]
defined, 45, [91]
diagnosis and, 13, [72]
ethics and, 37, [66, 84, 85, 86]
evaluation and, 24, 25, [77]
implementation and, 18, [75]
outcomes identification and, 14, [73]
planning and, 8, 16, [74]
professional practice evaluation and,
    [80, 81]
quality of practice and, [79, 80]
resource utilization and, [89, 90]
See also Education of patients and
    families; Patient
Financial issues. See Cost control

G

Generalist practice hospice and
    palliative nursing, 3–5, [65–68]
advocacy and ethics, 3–4, [66, 84]
assessment, 11, [71]
clinical judgment, 3, [66]
collaboration, 4, 35, [67, 86–87]
collegiality, 33, [82–83]
communication, 5, [67–68]
competencies, 3–5, [65–68]
consultation, 22, [76]
coordination of care, 20, [76]
cultural competence, 3, 4, [66, 67]
diagnosis, 13, [72]
education, 29, [81–82]
ethics, 37, [66, 84–85]
evaluation, 24, [77]
health teaching and health promotion,
    21, [76]
implementation, 18, [75]
leadership, 43
learning facilitation, 5, [67]
outcomes identification, 14, [73]
planning, 16, [74]
practice environment, 2, 5, 33, 42, 43,
    [65, 67, 81, 83, 87, 88]
prescriptive authority and treatment,
    23, [77]
professional practice evaluation, 31,
    [80–81]

professionalism, 4, [66]
quality of practice, 27–28, [79]
referral, [77]
research, 39, [87–88]
resource utilization, 41–42, [89]
roles, 3–6, [65–68]
systems thinking, 4, [67]
See also Advanced practice hospice
    and palliative nursing; Hospice
    and palliative nursing
Geriatric care, xi
health teaching and health promotion,
    21
See also Cultural competence
Guidelines
collaboration and, [87]
ethics and, [86]
leadership and, 44
outcomes identification and, 15
professional practice evaluation and,
    31
quality of practice and, 27, [79]
research and, [88]
See also Standards of practice;
    Standards of professional
    performance

H

Health teaching and health promotion
collaboration and, [87]
implementation and, 7, [75, 76]
standard of practice, 21, [76]
Healthcare policy, 4, [66]
education and, 29, [84]
ethics and, [86]
evaluation and, 24, 25
quality of practice and, 27, [79]
research and, 39, [88]
Healthcare providers
assessment and, 11, [71]
collaboration and, [86, 87]
collegiality and, [83]
defined, 45–46, [91]
diagnosis and, 13, [72]
evaluation and, 24
outcomes identification and, 14, [73]
planning and, [74]

Healthcare providers (*continued*)
quality of practice and, [80]
See also Collaboration; Interdisciplinary health care
Healthcare team. *See* Collaboration;
Interdisciplinary health care
Holistic care, 1, 11, [64]
Hospice Nurses Association (HNA), *xii*,
xiii, [63]
Hospice and Palliative Nurses Association
(HPNA), *xiii*, 7, [63, 69, 83]
Hospice and palliative nursing
activities, 1–2
body of knowledge, 4, 7, 14, 15, 17,
18, 23, 27, 28, 29, 30, 33, 39, 40,
[66, 68, 69, 71, 73, 74, 78, 80, 81,
88]
certification, *xi*, *xii*, *xiii*, 3, 6, 9, 28, 43,
[65, 68, 70, 80, 82]
characteristics, 1–2, [64–65]
cultural competence, 1, 2, 3, 4, 8, 14,
16, 17, 18, 21, 31, 37, [61, 64, 65, 67,
70, 73, 74, 75, 76, 82, 84]
education, *ix*, *x*, *xi*, 3, 5, 9, 29–30, 33,
35, 36, 39, 43, [60, 61, 65, 68, 70, 71,
79, 81–82, 83, 84, 85, 86, 87, 88]
ethics, *ix*, *xii*, 3–4, 9, 14, 18, 27, 37–38,
[60, 62, 66, 70, 75, 76, 82, 84–86]
goals, 1, [64]
healthcare providers and, 11, 13, 14,
24, 45–46, [71, 72, 73, 74, 80, 83, 86,
87, 91]
history, *x*–*xiii*, [60–63]
levels of practice, 3–6, [65–68]
practice environment, 2, [65]
roles, 3–6, [65–68]
scope of practice, 1–6, [64–68]
standards of practice, 7–8, 11–25,
[69–70, 71–78]
standards of professional
performance, 9, 27–44, [70, 79–90]
See also Advanced practice hospice
and palliative nursing; Generalist
practice hospice and palliative
nursing
Human resources. *See* Professional
development

I
Implementation, *xii*
collaboration and, [87]
defined, 46, [92]
evaluation and, 24
leadership and, 43
quality of practice and, 27, 28
standard of practice, 18–19, [75–77]
step in nursing process, 7, [69]
Information. *See* Data collection
Interdisciplinary health care, 1, 5, [64, 68]
assessment and, 11, 12
collaboration and, 35, 36, [67, 86, 87]
collegiality and, 33, 34, [83]
communication and, 5, [67]
coordination of care and, 20
defined, 46, [92]
diagnosis and, 13, [72]
education and, 5, [67, 82]
ethics and, 38, [85, 86]
evaluation and, 24, [77]
implementation and, 18, [75]
leadership and, 44
outcomes identification and, 14, [73]
planning and, 8, 16, 17, [74, 75]
professional practice evaluation and,
[81]
quality of practice and, 28, [79]
research and, [88]
resource utilization and, 41
See also Collaboration; Healthcare
providers
International Council of Nurses, *x*
Internet, 21
Interventions
health teaching and health promotion,
[76]
implementation and, [75]
planning and, 17, [74]
research and, [87]

J
Johns Hopkins Nursing Leadership
Academy for End-of-Life Care, [62]

K
Knowledge base. *See* Body of knowledge